Clinical
Health
Issues
Handbook

Karil Bellah, M.S., M.D.

Lawrence, Kansas

West Publishing Company

MINNEAPOLIS/ST. PAUL
NEW YORK
LOS ANGELES
SAN FRANCISCO

Acknowledgments

I am grateful to H. R. Fischer for her medical illustrations. I extend a special thanks to Linda Lyle, M.D., for her contribution to the glossary and input to the text.

K. B.

West's Commitment to the Environment

In 1906, West Publishing Company began recycling materials left over from the production of books. This began a tradition of efficient and responsible use of resources. Today, up to 95 percent of our legal books and 70 percent of our college and school texts are printed on recycled, acid-free stock. West also recycles nearly 22 million pounds of scrap paper annually—the equivalent of 181,717 trees. Since the 1960s, West has devised ways to capture and recycle waste inks, solvents, oils, and vapors created in the printing process. We also recycle plastics of all kinds, wood, glass, corrugated cardboard, and batteries, and have eliminated the use of styrofoam book packaging. We at West are proud of the longevity and the scope of our commitment to the environment.

Production, Prepress, Printing and Binding by West Publishing Company.

Illustration: Holly R. Fischer, M.F.A.
Composition: Atelier 88

Contents

CHAPTER 16

Urinary System   127

CHAPTER 17

Reproductive System   133

CHAPTER 18

Pregnancy and Development   143

CHAPTER 19

Prevention and Health Maintenance   151

Glossary   157

1 Introduction to Clinical Medicine

Each of us has had medical attention at some time. For some, it has been infrequent and has primarily involved preventive measures (such as immunizations or checkups). Others have made several visits to clinics or hospitals for more serious, ongoing health problems. In this supplemental clinical manual, pertinent health issues will be explored with the intent of providing you with information about certain common diseases. This manual is not intended to enable you to give medical advice to friends or family, but, instead, to answer general and specific questions you may have about health problems and give you a better understanding of clinical medicine.

First, let's examine what we mean by "disease." A *disease* is any disruption of the body's ability to function normally. Diseases can be caused by infections, can be the result of an injury, or can be due to an imbalance in the body's own regulatory mechanisms. Fortunately, the human body exhibits *adaptive responses* to diseases that enable it to heal or compensate for diseases. The extent of illness we experience is the result of the balance between disease and adaptation.

You certainly know by now that there are thousands of different diseases with a wide range of severity. Obviously, a common cold or a cut requiring stitches is not as severe or long-lasting as cancer or a heart attack. Thus, diseases can be described in different ways that indicate their character. In this respect, disease can be *minor* or *severe*. Depending on the duration, disease can be *acute* (short-term) or *chronic* (lasting a long time). Based on the extent of tissue or organ involvement, disease can be *local* (confined to one location or organ) or *systemic* (involving several organs throughout the body).

How do we know we are sick? Often we experience pain, a cough, an itch, or fatigue. *Symptoms* are alterations in sensation, appearance, or function that indicate illness. A symptom does not always tell us what disease we have (for example, a cough can be caused by pneumonia, cancer, or allergies) but certain diseases typically, but not always, cause the same symptoms. Do all diseases have symptoms? The answer is definitely no. High blood pressure is a very common "silent" disease leading to widespread health problems (stroke, heart attack, kidney disease); however, it is *asymptomatic* so that a person feels fine but in fact has a deadly disease. Other diseases, especially cancer, may be asymptomatic for long periods before symptoms become manifested. In contrast, the common cold is not a serious disease, but the symptoms are often debilitating.

Once we feel sick, we usually seek medical attention and see a healthcare professional, or *provider* (physician, nurse, or physician assistant). In addition to the symptoms, a *physical examination* is useful in determining what disease is the culprit. In a physical exam, a provider looks for certain changes from the norm in appearance, sound, or feel. For example, when you have a stomach ache, it could be from hepatitis or constipation. From inspecting the appearance of your abdomen, palpating (or touching) different areas of the abdomen, and listening to your bowel sounds with a stethoscope, the provider will usually differentiate the two problems.

Often, further medical studies or tests are needed to determine or confirm the diagnosis. The *diagnosis* of a disease is the recognition or determination of the nature of the disease based on the symptoms, physical exam, and specialized tests (if needed). In other words, it is identifying the disease (telling you your stomach ache is the disease called hepatitis). The other studies most often utilized in making a diagnosis are blood tests or radiographic studies (x-rays). In *blood tests*, an excess or deficiency of certain chemicals, blood cell types, hormones, and enzymes can be determined. For instance, you may feel very fatigued and look pale, and a blood test will show too few red blood cells or low iron. Now the diagnosis of anemia can be made. *X-rays* usually show structural changes like a broken bone (fracture) or an accumulation of infection in the lung (pneumonia). Not all diseases require a blood test or x-ray, but these studies are often helpful.

Once a diagnosis of a disease has been made, a plan to treat the disease is initiated. The *treatment* of a disease can be aimed either at curing the disease process or at alleviating the symptoms. Consider the symptom of blood in the urine with abdominal pain. If the diagnosis is a urinary tract infection, antibiotics can be given to destroy the bacteria causing the infection, thus curing the disease. If a kidney stone is the culprit, however, intravenous fluids and pain medications can be administered to decrease the symptoms, but the stone will usually pass on its own without a curative treatment.

The expected outcome of a disease can be estimated once the extent, duration, and severity of the illness are determined. The *prognosis* is an educated prediction of the outcome of the disease and potential complications associated with it. No prognosis can be exact because no human body is exactly like another, but usually the possibilities for recovery can be estimated, and generalizations about survival can be approximated.

How is medical information about a person recorded or reported to another health-care provider so that more input can be obtained? Usually, the patient's symptoms, physical exam, blood tests, and studies are prepared as a *case presentation*. In this way, the pertinent information can be consolidated in medical records and letters to other providers.

In this book, case presentations open each chapter to initiate thought about certain diseases related to a particular body system. These cases are merely examples of clinical entities and do not represent actual persons. Following the case presentation(s), a few questions will be asked, followed by brief discussions of the most common diseases affecting this system. We hope that you will find yourself answering many of the questions with the knowledge of human anatomy and human physiology you already have. Again, this is not intended to be a textbook to train medical professionals but is, rather, for your information about health and disease.

2 Integumentary System

CASE PRESENTATIONS

Molly, 7 years old, had just spent a week at day camp near the Lake of the Ozarks in Missouri. On the last day of camp, she noticed that her ankles were itching and started scratching them. Within a few hours, both her legs and arms were itching, and her camp leader noticed that she had a red rash covering her extremities. Molly felt well except for the itching, which was quite severe by this time. Her camp leader took her to see the camp nurse.

When the nurse examined Molly, he noticed a red, slightly raised rash on her ankles that was diffusely spread. On her legs and arms the rash was in a vertically streaked pattern that ended at her shorts and sleeves. Otherwise, he found Molly's exam to be normal.

The nurse told Molly she had *poison ivy* (a type of *contact dermatitis*) and gave her a cortisone cream to put on her rash and an antihistamine that she was to use for five days. He told her to stop scratching or the itching would become worse and spread all over her body. Over the next several days, the rash got better and in another week, Molly's skin was back to normal.

When Susan was a junior in high school, she developed a rash on her elbows and knees. The rash started in the winter and got better that summer. The rash did not itch, but it got red and burned when she took hot showers. It seemed to get worse again the next winter, but Susan did not worry about it because it did not hurt and she was able to cover it up with her winter clothes. When she started her freshman year of college, the rash became a lot worse, and when she was home that fall, she saw her family doctor.

Susan was taking no medications and had had all of her childhood immunizations. She did not smoke or drink alcohol and was not sexually active. She did not have any allergies.

A physical exam found an irregular, thick rash on her elbows and her knees, predominantly over the extensor tendons. The rash was very rough to the touch and appeared scaly and splotchy, mostly white with some reddish areas. Otherwise, her exam was normal.

Susan was told she had *psoriasis* and was started on therapy with topical (applied to the skin) medication and ultraviolet treatment. She is now 34 years old and still has to use these treatments to keep the rash under control. She has also developed a rash on her right wrist and has had problems with premature arthritis.

Questions

1. How are psoriasis and contact dermatitis different in symptoms, treatment, and duration?
2. Why did Susan's psoriasis flare when she started college?
3. Are all skin problems treated with topical medicine?
4. What agents cause skin problems?
5. Can you die from a skin disease?

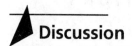

Discussion

Dermatology is the study of the skin and is the medical subspecialty that pertains to diseases of the skin. Over 60 million people in the United States bring skin disorders to the attention of a physician each year. Although few of these problems are curable, many are treatable, thus allowing at least symptomatic relief. Most dermatological disorders are primary diseases of the skin: however, some are manifestations of other systemic diseases. A few common primary skin disorders will be examined in the discussion below, but first let's consider dematological manifestations of other diseases.

Jaundice is a yellow discoloration of the skin that is caused primarily by liver disease. The skin itself is not diseased, but waste products that cannot be metabolized by the liver give the skin a yellow tinge. In other words, the abnormal skin is giving a clue that there is a problem affecting the liver. Because the skin is readily visible, the liver disease can be detected before other symptoms occur. Infections, cancers, and other diseases may be expressed in the skin, and most of the time the skin improves as the underlying disease is treated.

Dermatitis

A number of substances cause *dermatitis*. Contact dermatitis is an inflammatory reaction of the skin characterized by a red, itchy, rash that develops when a particular substance touches the skin. With poison ivy or poison oak, the "oil" on the leaves of the plant causes an immune, hypersensitivity reaction in the dermis, which draws antibodies and white blood cells into the area. The intensity of the rash depends on the total amount of contact and the amount of time the oil is on the skin. The oil can be spread to other parts of the body and to other people by direct contact. The reaction to the oil may be delayed for a couple of days after exposure to the plant, and it usually clears up in one to two weeks.

Contact dermatitis does not cause scarring, so treatment is aimed at relieving symptoms. Anti-inflammatory medication (like aspirin) can help the inflammation, and antihistamines are usually effective in relieving the itching. Also, wet compresses, baths, and topical drying lotions can offer relief. Topical steroidal preparations (cortisone creams or lotions) are potent anti-inflammatory agents and can be applied to severely affected areas. Prevention is the best "treatment" and involves seasonal avoidance of known culprits. If exposure occurs, immediate washing with water and soap alleviates the symptoms.

Other agents may cause dermatitis such as body soaps and lotions, detergents, fungus, talc and powders, chemicals, and urine or feces (diaper rash). Sometimes, agents such as medicine or food that are ingested may cause a rash or welts (*urticaria*). Urticaria often results from insect bites or stings as well.

Psoriasis

Psoriasis is a chronic skin disease that affects 1% to 3% of Americans. There is no identifiable cause of psoriasis, but there appear to be some genetic predispositions. Many factors exacerbate this condition, including infections, topical irritants, certain medications, and excessive sun. Psoriasis is primarily found on the knees, elbows, soles, palms, and scalp. The underlying disorder is an abnormality in keratinization of the epidermis (Figure 2.1), but some forms are accompanied by significant amounts of inflammation and pustule formation. These severe forms can be life threatening, but most cases can be controlled.

No cure is available for psoriasis, but symptomatic management can usually be achieved for most people through a variety of treatment modalities. Topical agents used for treatment include steroids, salicylic acid (an aspirin-like anti-inflammatory agent), coal tar, and anthralen (a cytotoxic agent). These agents can be used alone or in combination with other treatment regimens. Systemic steroids are not recommended for psoriasis because the side effects are such that long-term steroid use has significant risks. Methotrexate is a chemotherapeutic medication that inhibits DNA synthesis and is reserved for use in severe cases. Psoralen is a medication taken orally that makes the psoriatic skin more sensitive to ultraviolet radiation (UVA). Neither agent alone is effective, but a combined regimen (referred to as PUVA) is the most effective phototherapy available. Recently, a form of vitamin A has been found effective as a single oral agent in the treatment of psoriasis. Noticeable results take months and may be long lasting, but side effects limit its use.

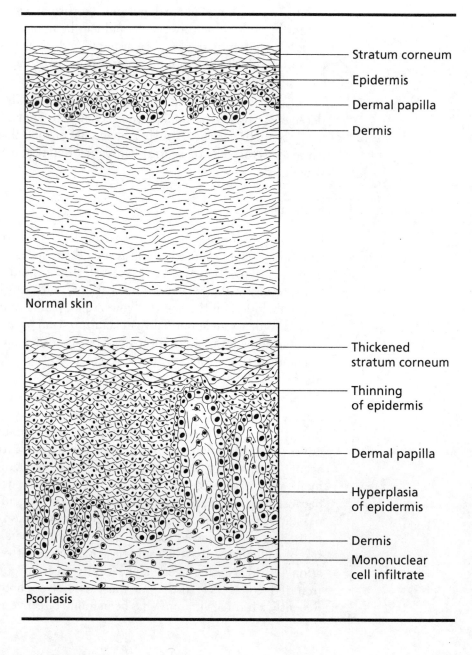

Figure 2.1
Histology of normal skin and of diseased skin in psoriasis. This disease results in thick, scaly patches.

Acne

Acne is a plague of teenagers and young adults. Acne is caused by the buildup of sebum (produced by sebaceous glands), bacteria, and dead cells, forming a plug in the hair follicles. When this "plug," or comedone (whitehead or blackhead) reaches the surface of the skin, it forms a pimple with the accompanying inflammation. These lesions typically form on the face, chest, upper back, and shoulders due to the high density of sebaceous glands in these areas. Acne first appears during puberty because the surging sex hormones affect the sebaceous glands. The natural course of acne is episodic, with clear periods between the outbreaks. Usually the lesions clear up, but in severe cases, deep cysts are formed that cause scarring.

The treatment of acne is diverse, and a regimen that works for one individual may not be effective in another. With the recent introduction of an oral vitamin A derivative, acne can be cured, but such a potent treatment is not needed in most individuals. Despite common belief, diet does not appear to play a significant role in the development of acne, nor do most cosmetics (although water-based cosmetics are better than oil based ones). The treatment of acne must be tailored to each person, but there are three basic modalities: topical care, antibiotics, and vitamin A derivatives.

Topical care may be appropriate for those with minimal pimples, whiteheads, and blackheads. Proper washing twice a day is beneficial, although no amount of washing is going to eliminate blackheads, since their formation has nothing to do with cleanliness. Topical preparations are of two types, comedolytics and antimicrobials. Comedolytics reduce the buildup of material in the hair follicles and actually help propel the sebum from the follicle. Tretinoin, or Retin-A, is currently available as a comedolytic. Topical antimicrobials, such as benzoyl peroxide, erythromycin, clindamycin, and meclocycline, work by decreasing the population of acne-causing bacteria. They are sometimes used in conjunction with tretinoin in order to augment the effects, but they should be applied at separate times as they will neutralize each other. Both topical forms of treatment will usually require 8 to 12 weeks before significant improvement is noted, as neither will have any effect on existing pimples.

Several oral antibiotics are effective when pustules and pimples are prominent. Again, time is needed to see a true effect of treatment, and for any given person it is impossible to predict which antibiotic will be most effective. If no response is seen in six weeks, another antibiotic is prescribed, and this pattern repeated until a successful agent is found.

Isotretinoin (an oral vitamin A derivative) does offer a cure for acne in 90% of persons who faithfully take it for 12 to 20 weeks. Accutane, the trade name, is most effective in cases of severe cystic acne. The most alarming side effects are severe birth defects in the babies of women taking the drug while pregnant. The danger of birth defects completely disappears if the medication is discontinued for several months prior to becoming pregnant.

Accutane can also cause an elevation in cholesterol and triglycerides in the blood, which can usually be controlled with diet modifications. Other annoying side effects are dry mouth and skin and increased susceptibility to sun damage. Despite these undesirable side effects, with close physician monitoring, isotretinoin offers a cure for severe acne and prevents permanent scarring and disfiguration that would otherwise result.

Infections

There are many skin infections, caused by a variety of infectious agents. We will examine three relatively common causes of skin infections—bacterial, fungal, and viral—but keep in mind that every type of infectious agent can involve the skin. Skin infections are difficult to manage in persons who are immunocompromised or who have AIDS, but most others can be effectively treated. Topical and systemic antibiotics are the mainstay of treatment for these annoying health problems.

Impetigo is a bacterial infection of the skin caused by staphylococcal and streptococcal organisms. The infection occurs primarily in children and appears as soft, honey-colored crusts on top of a red, weeping rash, but it may have a more blister-like appearance as well. Although the lesions may be found anywhere, they typically occur on the face, commonly under the nose, and may spread to surrounding skin or to distant areas. The infection is highly contagious, so bathing towels and clothes of the infected individual must be handled cautiously. Topical treatment with a new antibacterial ointment appears to be effective in minor cases, but the mainstay of treatment remains oral antibiotics. If scratching is kept to a minimum, the infection can be cleared without leaving any scars.

Gangrene is a more serious bacterial skin infection and can involve the deeper tissues if not treated promptly. This infection is more common in the extremities, in which the blood supply is poor, and if not aggressively treated, it may lead to amputation of the affected limb.

Fungal infections are among the most common skin afflictions and can occur at any location on the body. These infections are caused by five different types of fungi, some of which can involve hair follicles. In warm, moist areas on the body or after contact exposure with infected humans, dogs, or cats, fungi invade the stratum corneum, where they can multiply. This sets up a reaction in the dermis associated with itching and varying degrees of inflammation. The most common sites of infection are the feet (athlete's foot), the groin, the hands, and the nail beds. However, "ringworm" can occur anywhere on the body, including the scalp. The diagnosis of these characteristic rashes can be confirmed by scraping some scales from the borders of the lesions and examining for fungi under a microscope. A Woods light is a fluorescent light under which hair affected by certain types of fungi will appear yellow or green, but other types of fungi will be missed by this test. Cultures of the lesions may also be done, but these require several cultures and are less sensitive than direct microscopic examination. Treatment of fungal infections is determined by the extent and severity of the infection. Many topical antifungal creams and lotions are available over the counter. These are most effective when started soon after the rash begins. They should be applied twice a day to the lesions and the surrounding skin, and they should be continued for several days after it appears the rash is completely resolved to prevent chronic or recurrent infections. With athlete's foot, topical drying agents (aluminum chloride agents) prevent excessive sweating and can be extremely effective. Oral antifungal agents are reserved for widespread, progressive, or chronic infections and those involving the nail beds. The two oral agents currently available have provided effective treatment for many sufferers from this annoying problem, but long-term treatment and close attention to side effects are required. Topical steroids should be avoided, but antihistamines can usually provide some relief from itching.

Viral infections of the skin are common, diverse diseases that are difficult to treat; fortunately, most have a self-limiting course. Measles, chickenpox, and rubella (German measles) were once common childhood diseases, but measles and rubella are now less common. Just as smallpox has been eliminated with the adoption of a widespread vaccination program, the MMR vaccine (measles, mumps and rubella) has had a marked impact on these highly contagious diseases.

Despite these advances in preventing viral diseases, the most common virus affecting humans remains an enormous problem. The *herpes simplex virus* (HSV) causes very painful, blister-like lesions on an inflamed base that evolve to crusted lesions. The virus is shed from these lesions, is highly contagious, and is spread by direct contact. HSV has two characteristic distributions: 1) the oral mucosa and lips (canker sores and cold sores) and 2) the genitalia. Herpes is a sexually transmitted disease, and a very important fact to remember is that an infected person may be contagious even without evidence of the painful lesions.

HSV infections can be divided into three phases. The first phase is the primary (initial) infection. In addition to the extreme discomfort caused by the skin lesions, there is often accompanying fever, malaise, and locally tender lymph nodes. The skin lesions usually last one to two weeks but may persist for up to three weeks. When this phase resolves, the HSV becomes inactive and enters the latent phase. The virus remains dormant in the nerve root ganglion (collection of nerve cells) near the spinal cord that innervates the area of affected skin. It can survive here for years, even a lifetime. Under certain circumstances, it will travel down the nerve root and reinfect the skin resulting in the secondary (recurrent) phase. Infections, stress, fever, sunburn, menstruation, trauma, and dental work can trigger this secondary phase, but the mechanism is unclear. Typically, recurrent infections are less painful, do not produce fever and lymphadenopathy, and resolve in eight days. Unfortunately, the virus is in the skin approximately

48 hours prior to the outbreak and is shed in great numbers during this time. Only 50% of persons will have any hint that lesions are going to erupt, with the preceding symptoms of itching, burning, or pain. Again, this preceding stage (called the prodrome) is a highly contagious period, before lesions are apparent. The infection does not leave physical scars and is not fatal except in newborns and immunocompromised persons. There are other forms of HSV infections, such as those involving the central nervous system, but these are rare in the general population.

Treatment of the HSV has advanced over the years. There is no cure for genital herpes; thus, the thrust must be toward prevention with the use of condoms. Acyclovir is an antiviral agent that has been a breakthrough in the treatment of herpes. When applied topically, it reduces viral shedding and may offer some symptomatic relief. Oral acyclovir decreases symptoms, reduces viral shedding, and speeds healing in both initial and recurrent infections. It is most effective when initiated as early in the prodromal stage as possible. Acyclovir can also be taken at a lower dose on a daily basis to help prevent recurrent infections in those persons who have severe and frequent infections. Acyclovir does *not* prevent transmission of the HSV with sexual contact; thus, condoms must be used even with acyclovir.

Baldness

Baldness is a common form of hair loss, the cause of which is multifactorial. There is certainly a hereditary component in which males tend to follow the same pattern as their mother's father (maternal grandfather). Increased amounts of testosterone (and other "male" hormones) lead to baldness, as well as age.

In male pattern baldness, the hair on the top of the head is lost first, with a receding hairline around the face. The hair on the side of the head is largely preserved. This type of baldness is uncommon in women but may be caused by abnormal hormone production, malnutrition, iron deficiency, and thyroid problems.

Treatment of baldness is not required medically, but many people seek treatment for cosmetic reasons. A wide variety of "treatments" is available, but no oil, shampoo, lotion, vitamin, nutrient solution, or kelp extract will regenerate hair growth. Hair transplants are sometimes successful, and others are satisfied with certain hair weaving techniques. A topical ointment containing *minoxidil* (a medicine that was used to lower blood pressure) has offered new hope for some. When applied to the scalp two to three times a day for an indefinite length of time, hair growth increases in 30% to 50% of users at the end of one year of treatment. The treatment is expensive ($50 to $60 per month), and when treatment stops, balding recurs. There are also undesirable side effects on the cardiovascular system.

Ultraviolet Damage

Acute exposure to ultraviolet (UV) light causes sunburn. UV waves cause long-term skin damage as well, even in the absence of sunburn. Tanning and unnoticed sun exposure during outdoor activities contribute to wrinkles, leathery skin, and reddened, blotchy patches. Although these conditions are cosmetically disturbing, they pose no real health threat. However, UV exposure also causes precancerous and cancerous skin lesions. These cancers are caused by the transformation of epidermal cells into malignant ones and can present important health problems.

Two types of UV light cause skin damage, long-wave A (UVA) and midrange sunbeam (UVB). UVB, emitted from the sun, is quite intense and is responsible for the damage to skin caused by the sun. However, UVA has become increasingly common as a cause of ultraviolet-related skin problems with the introduction of tanning salons. Tanning salons once primarily used lamps that emitted UVB waves, but most have converted to UVA lamps, advertised as "safer than the sun." This claim is not true, as UVA penetrates deeper into the skin than UVB. This penetration creates problems by damaging deep blood vessels, burning the cornea of the eye, and worsening sunburns caused by UVB. In addition, the UVB-related problems (skin wrinkling and cancer) are caused by UVA as well, and they may be worse when caused by UVA than when caused by the sun.

The best "treatment" for UV damage (both acute sunburn and long-term skin aging and cancer) is prevention. Unfortunately, no sunscreens are ideal, because they are not fully resistant to water and sweat and must be reapplied frequently. Para-amino benzoic acid (PABA) sunscreens are more water- and sweat-resistant than other types because they interact with the keratin in the stratum corneum.

Skin Cancer

Skin cancers are quite common and usually quite curable. (The exception is malignant melanoma, discussed below.) Solar radiation (sun exposure) is the single greatest risk factor for developing skin cancer. Genetic factors are also important, with fair-skinned, light-eyed individuals, especially those of Northern European origin, having the greatest predisposition to develop skin cancer.

The two skin cancers that are usually not life-threatening are *basal cell epithelioma* (BCE) and *squamous cell carcinoma* (SCC). Both are locally invasive but rarely spread elsewhere in the body. BCE typically occurs as a pearly nodule on the central areas of the face. SCC is found on the face, arms, and back of the hands and appears as a rapidly growing red nodule that may ulcerate and bleed. Red scaly flat spots in these areas are usually precancerous and are treated before they become a cancer. Once the cancer appears, it is removed by excision (cutting) or by electrical burning and scraping. Topical medicines are used to treat precancerous lesions. Once removed, the cancer is cured, but there is high risk of developing new cancers, and close follow-up is needed.

Malignant melanoma is a potentially fatal skin cancer that arises from the pigment-producing cells in the skin, the melanocytes. It is important to recognize the four characteristic features of malignant melanoma and to check your own skin and that of family members, as early detection and treatment of this cancer markedly improve survival (Figure 2.2). The lesions look like moles with the following features: 1) raised surface, 2) irregular borders, 3) dark and nonuniform color, and 4) apparent growth. Melanoma may arise on either sun-exposed or unexposed areas of the body and may appear as new lesions or arise from a pre-existing mole. The most important risk factor is solar radiation, and severe sunburn in childhood greatly increases the chance of developing this cancer. Genetic factors probably also play a role.

Early detection and treatment by excision are crucial, as this cancer can spread throughout the body and cause fatal complications, commonly bleeding. If the cancer is removed when it is small and contained within the skin, the survival rate is 90%, but if it has already spread throughout the

FIGURE 2.2
Melanoma on the posterior thigh. A raised lesion with an irregular border and nonuniform color is suspicious for melanoma, especially if it is growing.

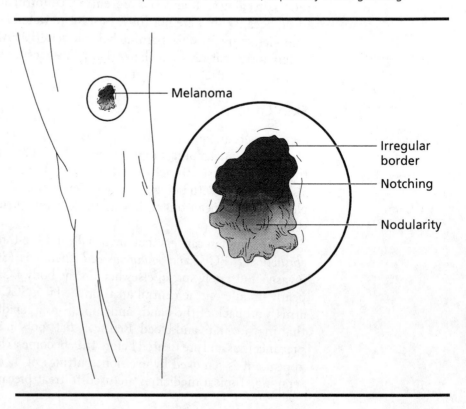

body, it is almost always fatal. Radiation and chemotherapy are not very effective treatments for malignant melanoma.

The sun damage that increases the risk of cancer can begin in early childhood, and much of the damage is already done by the age of 18 years. It is very important for all persons to wear sunscreens and protective clothing, including hats, while in the sun.

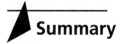 **Summary**

Diseases of the skin receive attention largely because they are readily visible. Pain, itching, and burning are common symptoms which also prompt persons with dermatological diseases to seek medical attention. Unfortunately, skin cancers are not symptomatic, and melanoma (the skin cancer with the greatest mortality) frequently occurs on parts of the body not easily seen. Symptomatic treatment is possible for most skin diseases; however, complete cure may not always be achieved.

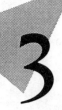

Skeletal System

CASE PRESENTATION

Mrs. Anderson is a busy, sharp 80-year-old who lives alone in a small town. When she was 12 years old, she fell out of a barn loft on the farm where she grew up but was not seriously injured. Four weeks ago, she was visiting her neighbor, and when she left, she stumbled down three porch steps. Immediately she had pain in her left hip and could not move her left leg. When her neighbor tried to help her up, Mrs. Anderson could not support her own weight. The emergency medical team was called and took her to the hospital by ambulance.

Mrs. Anderson has a history of high blood pressure and takes one medicine for this problem. She does not smoke and does not drink alcohol. After the accident her blood pressure was normal, but her heart rate was slightly increased. Her physical exam was normal except her left leg was found to be an inch shorter than her right, and her foot was rotated outward (externally rotated).

An x-ray of her left hip showed a fracture of the neck of the femur, and the bone's shaft was displaced behind the head. Laboratory tests revealed a low red blood cell count.

She was given medication for the pain and admitted to the hospital. Later that day, an orthopedic surgeon operated on her fractured femur and inserted a metal plate to stabilize the bone. Three days later, Mrs. Anderson started walking in physical therapy, and she went home a week later but had to use a walker to get around.

Questions

1. Why did Mrs. Anderson break her hip stumbling down a few steps, whereas, at 12, she had fallen a great distance and had not been hurt?
2. What symptoms did Mrs. Anderson experience?

3. How did the physical exam and x-ray aid in the diagnosis?
4. What did the surgeon do that allowed Mrs. Anderson a speedy recovery?

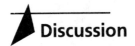

Discussion

The skeletal system is the supporting structure of the body. Although many disorders affect the bones, the most common are fractures, osteoporosis (thinning of the bones), and cancer. *Orthopedic surgeons* are physicians who specialize in problems affecting the bone, joints, and musculature. Although their title connotes the need for some type of surgery, several orthopedic injuries do not require surgical intervention. Often these injuries will heal with proper care and physical rehabilitation. *Physiatrists* are physicians who specialize in rehabilitation, and *physical therapists* are primarily involved with supervising and delivering the treatments. Many doctors and physician assistants are well trained in orthopedic medicine and often cast broken bones, treat athletic injuries, and prescribe physical therapy. However, only a small percentage of orthopedic problems require surgery for proper healing.

Fractures

Bone fractures are caused by trauma or may result from the thinning of bones in osteoporosis. Fractures are diagnosed by clinical presentation and x-rays, which may show the obvious discontinuity of the bone or may show a faint line of disruption of the cortex (outer layer) of the bone. Some fractures are visible to the eye, because the broken bone penetrates the skin. This usually occurs with severe injuries such as car accidents. Other fractures, caused by overuse (stress fractures), can be detected only with specialized "bone scans." Fractures are classified according to the extent of discontinuity and according to whether the two broken ends are in contact, penetrate the skin, are shattered, or overlap (Figure 3.1). The treatment for a fracture (such as immobilization, casting, surgery, or metal support devices) is determined by the type of fracture, but the healing process is the same for all fractures.

After a bone has been broken, the first step in the healing process is the formation of the *procallus* by the blood clot that organizes around the fractured segments. (Bone tissue has a good blood supply, which is very important in healing; because of this plentiful blood supply, however, there can be a good deal of blood loss when a bone is broken.) The procallus later develops connective tissue and cartilage and is called the *callus*. The callus effectively immobilizes the fracture site. Finally, the callus calcifies, and bone remodeling begins.

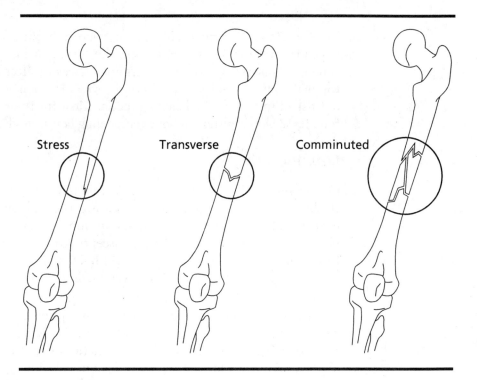

FIGURE 3.1
Three types of fractures of the femur. It is obvious that a comminuted fracture will require casting and probably metal support (pins or plates) for proper healing. In contrast, a stress fracture will heal nicely if overuse is avoided.

Immobilization of the fracture site is critical for proper healing and can be achieved in several ways, depending on the extent and type of fracture. In some instances, splinting may be adequate (such as with a finger). Casting is the most common means of immobilization. The location of the cast and the position of the bone and joint(s) in the cast are such as to relieve stress on the bone. For example, a fracture of the radius requires casting of the wrist joint to ensure adequate healing. Surgery may also be required either to realign the bone segments or to attach metal plates or pins to the bone that immobilize and strengthen the fracture site. In some cases, the metal plates or pins can be removed after the fracture has healed.

In some cases, the bone does not reunite and form a callus so there is no mechanism for bone remodeling to occur. When this happens, a *bone graft* can be used by taking living bone from elsewhere in the body (usually the iliac crest) and attaching it to the fracture site. Sometimes a mixture of crushed bone and fluids can be used to make a *bone patch* to promote healing. Finally, electrical currents may also prove to be beneficial in bone healing by stimulating new bone growth.

The amount of time required for fracture healing varies widely and depends on the type of fracture and the means of immobilization. The extent of bone healing can be determined by x-rays after the callus begins to calcify. These studies help determine when the bone can be used without risk of impairing the healing process. Most fractures are immobilized for 4 to 12 weeks, although bone remodeling continues beyond this time.

Osteoporosis

Osteoporosis is the loss of bone mass, commonly thought of as thinning of the bones. It is an asymptomatic disease affecting millions of people, especially the elderly, and is more common in women than men. Osteoporotic bones are thinner, weaker, and more susceptible to fracture, even if there is little or no trauma. The consequences of fracture are usually severe, resulting in hospitalization, surgery, and even increased risk of dying.

Osteoporosis is caused by osteoclast activity outpacing osteoblast activity, with the net result being bone reabsorption. Several factors influence the rate and extent of reabsorbtion and bone loss. In general, bone resorbtion predominates over bone formation after the age of 35 years, approximately, so that you begin losing bone. Obviously, if you are a "big-boned" person, you can afford to lose more bone mass before reaching the critical stage at which there is an increased risk of fracture. Likewise, if you have "small bones" to start with, you will be at that critical stage sooner. Therefore, both *age* and *body build* will influence your chance of developing osteoporosis. *Bone stress* is also important because your bones are stimulated to grow if they are being stressed by weight or muscular activity. Very thin people and inactive people are more prone to develop osteoporosis than heavier, active ones. *Estrogen* (a "female" hormone) plays a protective role in preventing bone loss. Thus, when a woman enters menopause and her body stops producing estrogen, there is accelerated bone loss. Finally, other factors such as smoking, alcohol use, poor dietary habits, and hereditary factors also contribute to osteoporosis.

Before resulting in a fracture, osteoporosis can be diagnosed by an x-ray, usually of the wrist or spine. The bones appear thinned, and decreased bone content can be determined by comparing the density of the bone with a standard scale. This measurement of bone density is clinically useful for detection of osteoporosis, but treatment is usually less effective once this bone loss has occurred. As you will see below, prevention is the most effective way to deal with the complications of osteoporosis, especially fractures.

The most common sites of fractures in osteoporosis are the spine, wrist, and hip. Compression fractures of the vertebrae are caused by everyday stress and usually the bones gradually collapse from the weight of the body (Figure 3.2). When this occurs, the normal curve of the spine is lost, and a person develops a concave curve and appears hunched over. Wrist

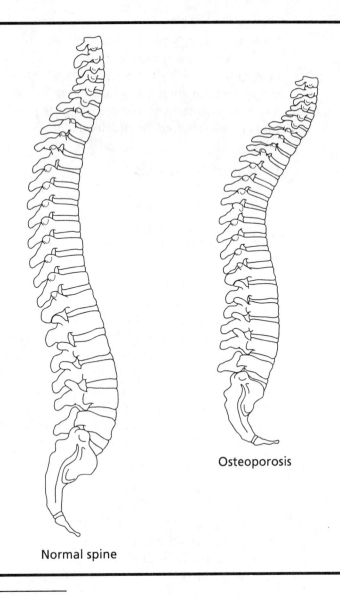

Osteoporosis

Normal spine

FIGURE 3.2
Normal spine and spine in osteoporosis. Notice the compression of the vertebrae and marked curvature of the osteoporotic spine.

fractures are common because the radius and ulna are narrow bones and because one uses a hand to break a fall. Hip fractures are the most serious fractures, especially in the elderly. Rarely does full motion return to the joint, and many will need some type of walking assistance.

The best treatment of osteoporosis is prevention of bone loss. This can be achieved by three important measures. First, it is important to have a proper *diet* with adequate amounts of calcium and Vitamin D. This is true during childhood and into old age to maintain proper bone balance.

Second, regular, weight-bearing *exercise* increases bone mass. Unfortunately, swimming and cycling do not offer as much protection as walking or jogging. Finally, *estrogen* replacement in women who have had their ovaries removed by surgery or who are entering menopause helps prevent bone loss. It is important to address the issue of estrogen therapy with healthcare providers before too much bone mass is lost.

Cancer of the Bones

Bone cancer can be divided into two major groups: 1) *primary* bone cancers, which originate from bone tissues, and 2) *metastatic* cancer, in which cancer from another organ (the lung, for example) metastasizes (spreads) to the bone.

Primary bone cancers usually grow quickly and spread very rapidly which often makes treatment very difficult. The symptoms associated with bone cancer are pain and swelling, but often it is asymptomatic until a fracture occurs at the site of the cancer. The cancer can usually be detected with x-rays or CAT scans and a bone biopsy is needed to make the diagnosis. In a bone biopsy, a piece of bone tissue is removed and processed for analysis under a microscope. In most cases, the cancer must be removed with surgery, sometimes resulting in an amputation. Often chemotherapy or radiation therapy is needed to further treat the disease. The chance of survival with bone cancer depends on whether the entire tumor can be removed before it spreads.

Metastatic bone lesions are very common with other types of cancers, especially those of the lung, breast, kidney, thyroid, and prostate. Once a cancer has spread to the bones, the hope for cure diminishes because it is very difficult to rid the bone of the malignant cells. Sometimes chemotherapy and radiation therapy can be given to decrease the pain associated with bone metastases.

Bone Infections

Infections in the bones are rare but occur most commonly in persons with diabetes mellitus and atherosclerosis (hardening of the arteries) in the lower extremities. Usually, there is a sore or ulcer on the skin over the bony infection that has not healed over a long period. An x-ray of the infected bone does not detect the infection until it has reached an advanced stage. For early detection, a bone scan, CAT scan, or even more specialized studies are required. Once the infection has been diagnosed, treatment with antibiotics must be given for several weeks (usually six weeks). If the infection cannot be cured, however, an amputation may be needed so that the infection does not spread and jeopardize more tissue.

Amputations

An *amputation* is the removal of an external body part such as a toe or arm. Sometimes a traumatic amputation is the result of an injury from an automobile or farming accident. Surgical amputations are used therapeutically for the treatment of some bone cancers or infections or when there is a lack of oxygen (in the blood) reaching an extremity, as in hardening of the arteries. Sometimes an injury may be so severe that the limb cannot be repaired, and an amputation is done. *Phantom pain* is the sensation of pain or feeling in a limb that has been removed because the brain still receives signals from the nerves that previously innervated the extremity. This sensation usually goes away over time. A *prosthesis* is an artificial body part that can replace the one amputated. A great deal of technology has been invested in making prostheses functional.

Marfan's Syndrome

Marfan's syndrome is an inherited disease of the collagen fibers in the body. The most obvious abnormalities involve the skeletal system and include tall stature, long limbs and digits, chest and spine deformities, and lax joints. These skeletal problems rarely lead to any significant medical problems, but they are used to detect the disease. Persons with Marfan's syndrome have visual problems due to changes in the lens of the eye or the length of the eyeball. The most alarming problems involve leaky valves of the heart or an aorta that may rupture without any warning. Many affected persons undergo valve replacement or repair of the aorta before a catastrophic event can occur.

Acromegaly

After puberty, the growth plates in the bones close and growth stops. If there is overproduction of the growth hormone (which stimulates bones to grow) later in life, certain bones in the face, hands, and feet will enlarge. This condition is called *acromegaly.* Acromegaly is suspected when a person has changed hat size or shoe size and is confirmed by x-raying the affected bones and measuring the amount of growth hormone.

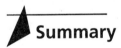

Summary

Bone diseases and injuries are problematic because movement and mobility are hindered. Bone fractures require immobilization to allow healing to take place. Immobilization can be achieved by a variety of techniques but casting is the most common. Osteoporosis is quite prevalent in the elderly and accounts for significant medical, emotional, economic, and social burdens in this population. Prevention of this disease begins in early adulthood with proper dietary habits and adequate exercise to build and maintain bone mass.

4 Articulations

CASE PRESENTATIONS

Ted, Jr., was an active college student without any medical problems. One Saturday, he was playing a game of touch football and was knocked from the side on his right thigh. He fell to the ground and instantly felt a knife-life pain in his right knee. When he got up to walk, his knee felt unstable and kept locking on him. His teammates had to help him back to the dorm, and he borrowed a pair of crutches to ambulate. The next day, his knee was swollen and very painful. He went to see the sports medicine doctor at the student health center.

On examination, the right knee was red and warm to the touch. There was a large joint effusion (excess fluid collection in the joint bursa), and his knee was very tender to the touch. There was a mild amount of pain when the knee was supported and not moving, but any amount of movement increased the pain, and Ted, Jr., could not move his knee freely. When the doctor examined the knee, the joint was stable, but passive movement produced pain. When the doctor flexed and extended the knee, there was a popping sound in the joint. This movement nearly sent Ted off the exam table with pain.

An x-ray of the knee did not show any fractures, but a large joint effusion was seen. The doctor "tapped" Ted's knee, removing a moderate amount of fluid (a joint aspiration), and Ted felt much better. The doctor put a splint on Ted's knee, told him to use crutches and not put weight on the knee, instructed him to keep ice on the knee, and made an appointment for him to see an orthopedic surgeon.

The orthopedic surgeon performed arthroscopy (looking into the joint with a small fiber-optic scope) on Ted's knee. He told Ted he saw a tear of the lateral meniscus. The surgeon then performed arthroscopic surgery and shaved off the torn cartilage. After Ted spent a few weeks in physical therapy, his knee was back to normal.

Ted, Sr., 56 years old, had intermittent pain and stiffness in his knees and hips. His pain was worse at the end of the day and sometimes when he came home from his job as a truck loader, he could barely walk. Rarely, he noticed a swollen knee joint and sometimes his knees locked. His doctor took an x-ray and told Ted, Sr., that "wear and tear" arthritis was affecting his joints. The doctor put him on a medication similar to aspirin to decrease the pain. Unfortunately, his right knee became so painful that he could not work. He had a surgical replacement of the knee joint with a metal prosthesis. After physical rehabilitation, Ted had much less pain and more range of motion in his right knee.

Questions

1. How did the onset of symptoms differ between Ted and his father?
2. What can an x-ray show about a joint, and what can't it show?
3. What are the differences between arthroscopic surgery and a joint replacement?
4. What other disorders can affect the joints?

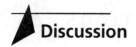

Discussion

Joint disorders may be caused by injuries, overuse, or systemic diseases. In all of these problems, any part or parts of the joint may be involved. *Arthritis* means inflammation of the articulations, regardless of the cause. Some joint diseases are limited to the joints themselves, but in other syndromes, arthritis is just one manifestation of a disease process that occurs in other parts of the body as well. *Arthralgia* means pain in the articulations, which may occur without inflammation. For example, sometimes you can suffer from aching joints when you have the flu or a cold. There is no inflammation in the joints, but you feel pain. A *rheumatologist* is a physician primarily concerned with diseases of the joints, other connective tissues in the body, and the immune system. The following discussion will address joint injuries, arthritis, and treatments.

Dislocations

Nearly everyone has had a joint dislocation at some time. Dislocations are not serious injuries, and most of them relocate without any intervention. Dislocations are almost always caused by trauma or excessive use. Commonly dislocated joints are fingers, toes, elbows and shoulders. (Dislocations of knees and hips are much less common and are usually caused by automobile accidents.) When a finger or toe joint becomes displaced, the tendons and ligaments surrounding the joint usually act to "pop" the joint back into place. With elbows and shoulders, gentle traction is used to realign the bones. Even with the joint back in place, swelling, pain, and stiffness may persist for several days.

X-rays are often taken when a joint is dislocated to make sure there is not a fracture. Fractures involving joints are often serious and don't heal well. When a joint is dislocated, the tendons and ligaments are stretched, which makes it easier for the joint to be dislocated again. This is especially true with the shoulder, which can become dislocated with easy throwing actions. Persons who frequently dislocate their shoulders may learn how to get them back into place, saving themselves a trip to the clinic or emergency room.

Bursitis

Bursitis is a common problem in which the bursae become inflamed. A bursa is a sac, filled with synovial fluid, that serves as a buffer in areas of friction in the body, especially around joints. There are approximately 150 bursae in the body, all of which are subject to inflammation. The cause of bursitis is usually injury or repetitive use, but arthritic joints may also have bursitis. The symptoms are pain, which often limits movement, and swelling. Sometimes bursitis is caused by infection and can be serious. Bursitis frequently involves the elbow, shoulder, or knee.

Treatment of bursitis involves immobilizing the areas of friction around the bursa. This is usually done by splinting. Moist heat applied to the area for 20 minutes several times a day assists healing, and anti-inflammatory drugs (similar to aspirin) should be taken for two weeks. If this regimen is not effective, the bursa can be injected with a local pain killer.

Arthroscopic Surgery

Arthroscopic (*arthro* = joint, *scopic* = scope) surgery has emerged in the past several years as an alternative to joint surgery for diagnosis and treatment of certain injuries. The technique of arthroscopic surgery involves making a small incision into the joint to insert a flexible, fiber-optic scope, which allows visualization of the joint structures. Another incision is made on the other side of the joint to insert surgical instruments, which can be used to repair or remove damaged tissue(s) in the joint. This procedure can be done with local or general anesthesia but usually does not require hospitalization and is less traumatic than joint surgery. Arthroscopic surgery has been used most frequently for repair of the knee joint but can be used for the elbow, wrist, and ankle also.

Artificial Joints

Replacements of the hip, knee, and other joints have become some of the most commonly performed surgical procedures, with an estimated half a million people receiving artificial joints each year. Since the advent of artificial joints in the 1960s, this technique has offered millions of people relief from the pain and decreased mobility associated with advanced stages of arthritis and other diseases affecting the joints. Although hip and knee replacements are the most common, techniques have been developed for artificial shoulder, wrist, elbow, and finger joints.

An artificial joint is designed to imitate the structure of the native joint. In the hip, the acetabulum is fitted with a metal "cup," into which a "ball" attached to a metal shaft is placed (Figure 4.1). The metal shaft is then inserted into the femur, which has the femoral head removed at the neck. These two metal pieces are then "cemented" to the respective bones with an acrylic bone cement. (Recent advances have developed metal devices that do not require cement; instead, native bone grows into the device to fit it to the bone.) The supportive structures of the joint remain intact, but the stability and mobility of the artificial joint never equal those of a healthy joint. Knee replacements are performed in much the same way as hip replacements. In knee replacements, an artificial patellar "button" may be inserted.

Functional use of an artificial joint can be expected for 10 to 15 years after surgery. Most joints "fail" after this time because of loosening of the

FIGURE 4.1

Osteoarthritis of the hip and hip replacement with artificial joint. When the femoral head and acetabulum become eroded, a hip replacement is needed. The prosthetic acetabular "cup" and femoral head are "cemented" into place to provide a metallic joint surface.

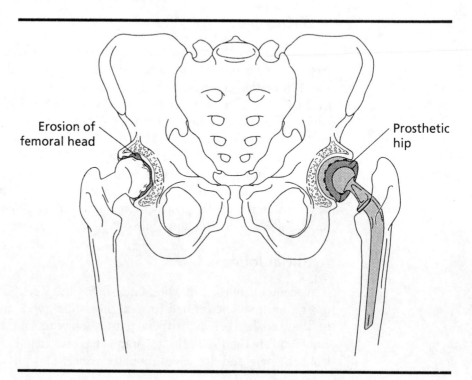

Erosion of femoral head

Prosthetic hip

components from the native bone. In most cases, another replacement operation can be performed. Bone fractures around the artificial joint and infections can also cause complications, usually necessitating another surgery. Although joint replacement is not the only surgical treatment for severe joint diseases, it is used extensively, and few complications arise in the hands of experienced orthopedic surgeons,

Joint Aspirations and Injections

Joint aspiration means the removal of synovial fluid from the joint cavity. Excess fluid in the joint cavity is removed by inserting a needle into the joint space and withdrawing the fluid through a syringe. This is both a diagnostic procedure, as the fluid can be analyzed to determine what is causing the joint problem, and a therapeutic procedure, as aspiration of the excess fluid can markedly decrease pain and improve movement. In some diseases and injuries, a local painkiller like xylocaine (often used for dental work) can be *injected* into the joint, usually through the same needle used to do the aspiration. If a more potent medicine is needed, a cortisone-like drug can also be injected into the joint. This will usually alleviate pain for several months.

Sprains

A *sprained joint* is one in which the injury has resulted in a complete or partial tear of the ligament(s) or tendon(s) supporting the joint structure. Often, the joint capsule is also injured, as well as cartilage. If the force of the injury is great, the ligament or tendon may tear a piece of bone away from the joint, resulting in an *avulsion fracture*. X-rays are needed to detect a fracture, but they cannot show the sprained ligaments or tendons.

The treatment of sprains depends on the severity of the injury, whether the joint structure is stable, and whether the joint is weight-bearing. Initially, rest, ice, elevation, and wrapping with an elastic bandage will reduce the swelling and pain. Aspirin-like medications are also quite effective at reducing the inflammation. If the sprain is severe, casting for immobilization and crutches for up to six weeks may be needed to ensure proper healing.

Slipped Discs

Lower back pain is a common problem among Americans and is responsible for vast numbers of dollars in worker's compensation and missed work. Slipped discs are responsible for much of the pain as well as for many non-work-related back problems. Over time the annulus fibrosus between the vertebral bodies weakens from everyday use (against gravity) and exertion related to lifting. The nucleus pulposus is under a lot of stress transmitted through the axial skeleton. This stress ruptures the annulus, causing the nucleus to protrude into the annulus and, often, into the vertebral canal (Figure 4.2). This can occur acutely with lifting, bending, coughing, or sneezing, or it may develop gradually with no recollection of a specific injury. The disc spaces above and below the fifth lumbar vertebrae are by far the most commonly affected, and it is unusual to have a slipped disc in another location. A "herniated" disc is quite painful and severely limits motion of the spine. The nucleus may protrude to impinge on the spinal cord or the nerves, a condition that requires urgent medical attention. Most herniated discs heal with rest and medication, but surgery is sometimes required to relieve the pain or neurological damage.

Arthritis

Arthritis, as you have seen, denotes the inflammation of a joint. An inflamed joint causes pain, stiffness, and swelling. Arthritic joints are often red and nearly always hurt more with movement than at rest. If the arthritis is severe and progressive, joint deformities may develop, and the disease may become crippling. In the following discussion, the three most common causes of arthritis will be considered, although there are certainly many more less common causes.

FIGURE 4.2
Herniated disc. The nucleus pulposus has protruded through the annulus and into the neural foramen. The resulting impingement on the nerve root leads to neurological symptoms.

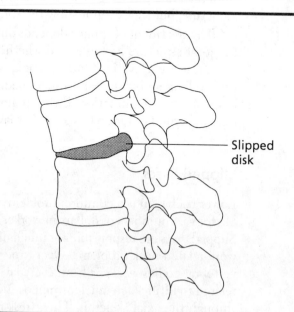

Slipped disk

Osteoarthritis is the "wear and tear" arthritis that occurs with the degeneration of the joints with age. The knees and hips are most commonly affected by this type of arthritis, but it can involve the joints in the upper extremities, especially in the hands. The cause is not known, but the disease is more common in women, in obese individuals, and in joints that have previously been injured or overused. Athletic activity does not increase the risk of developing osteoarthritis unless an injury occurs. The treatment of osteoarthritis involves aspirin-like medications to decrease the inflammation and an exercise program (physical rehabilitation) to preserve or increase joint mobility. If the disease progresses and becomes severely painful, with a decreased ability to ambulate, a joint replacement may be indicated.

Rheumatoid arthritis is an *autoimmune disorder* in which a confused immune system attacks the body's own tissues. Unlike the degenerative process of osteoarthritis, with rheumatoid arthritis there is a buildup of inflamed joint tissue that eventually destroys the joint. Rheumatoid arthritis is usually symmetrical, affecting the same joints on each side of the body, and is more common in the neck and the upper extremities, especially the small joints of the hand and wrist. The cause of this debilitating disease is not known, but there appear to be hereditary factors. As with osteoarthritis, medication and exercise are important in the treatment of rheumatoid arthritis. Also, gold, drugs used against malaria, and some anticancer medications have been effective at stopping the progression of the arthritis. Again, as a last resort, a joint replacement may be needed.

Gout is an acute arthritis, unlike osteoarthritis and rheumatoid arthritis, which develop over a long period. Gout typically affects the joints in the feet, especially the big toe, and comes on suddenly, causing excruciating pain, redness, and swelling. In gout, metabolic substances in the body form "crystals" in the joint space, and when the body reacts by sending in immune cells to get rid of the crystals, an impressive inflammatory process occurs. The crystals do not cause the pain, but rather the body's own cells are the culprits. Once an attack of gout occurs, treatment is directed at decreasing the effects of the immune cells. Prevention is a better approach, and medications are available to prevent the crystals from forming in the first place.

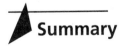 **Summary**

Arthritis is the inflammation of a joint(s) which has many causes. Rheumatoid arthritis and osteoarthritis progress to cause joint destruction or crippling joint deformities and may necessitate a joint replacement. Short of these outcomes, oral medications and medications injected into the joint offer relief from pain and stiffness. Joint injuries are common among active persons but with appropriate care and precaution, full recovery can usually be expected.

5 Musculature

CASE PRESENTATION

Joe, 21 years old, was a member of his college's cross-country team. In his junior year he was plagued by a charley horse in his left calf that bothered him off and on toward the end of the season. Even so, he was able to finish the season and recorded good times. In his senior year Joe made a real effort to work on his left calf and paid special attention to warming it up and stretching it before his training runs. During the second week of practice, he was running across a field and hit a ditch, landing very hard and off balance on his right foot. He immediately felt pain in his right calf, and although he could stand, he was unable to walk without severe pain and limping.

He was helped back to campus and saw the trainer. His right calf was flaccid, painful, and swollen. He was unable to extend his foot, and although he was able to flex his foot, it caused pain. The trainer sent Joe for a x-ray, which did not show a fracture. But when he was evaluated by an orthopedist, Joe was told he had ruptured his Achilles tendon. Initially his ankle was splinted, but the following day he underwent surgical repair of the tendon and was in a cast for the remainder of the cross-country season.

Questions

1. What is a "charley horse"?
2. Why was Joe unable to finish the season with a torn tendon but could run with a charley horse?
3. What are some common athletic injuries?
4. What other diseases affect the muscles?

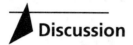

Discussion

Muscle injuries are quite common among all age groups. Basically, they can be divided into two broad categories: 1) those that result from acute traumatic injury and 2) those that occur from overuse of the muscle or muscle groups. Muscle injuries largely affect active, athletic individuals, "weekend athletes" (those who live sedentary lives but overdo it on a weekend), and people who perform repetitive motions at their jobs, such as typists or manual laborers. Usually, the injuries are minor and resolve without serious complications; however, surgery sometimes may be needed to restore proper function and relieve pain.

There are very few *primary muscle diseases*. The main one is muscular dystrophy, which will be discussed below. Other diseases that involve the muscles, such as cerebral palsy or polio, attack the nervous system but are most evident because of their effect on the muscles. These will be discussed in other chapters. Still other diseases affect the neuromuscular junction. One example of a neuromuscular disease is *myasthenia gravis*, in which the body produces antibodies that attack the acetylcholine receptors. *Botulism* is a form of food poisoning in which bacteria release poisons that prevent the release of acetylcholine from the nerve terminals and may result in paralysis or even death.

Muscle Cramps

A charley horse is another name for a *cramp* or *spasm* in a muscle. Muscle cramps are very painful, come on suddenly, and may cause the muscle to knot up and twitch. Muscle cramps usually occur after exercise or during sleep and are relieved by stretching or massaging the painful muscle. The cramp usually lasts only minutes and no permanent damage is done to the muscle or surrounding structures. The exact cause of muscle cramps is not known, but poor blood flow to the muscle and the accumulation of lactic acid or other chemicals in the muscle probably play a role. Unfortunately, the replacement of neither salt, potassium, nor other ions decreases the risk of cramps, but good conditioning with careful warm up and cool down activities may prevent muscle cramps.

Compartment Syndrome

The *anterior compartment* of the lower limb contains the tibialis anterior muscle and other muscles that dorsiflex the foot. These muscles are extensively used in sports requiring running, and they hypertrophy in proportion to their use. These muscles, like others in the body, are confined within their fascia, a sheath of connective tissue. This connective tissue is composed mostly of collagenous fibers and contains few elastic fibers; thus, it is relatively inelastic. When the muscles within the anterior compartment hypertrophy rapidly, they become entrapped and compressed within their compartment of fascia, which cannot distend to allow for the increasing muscle mass (Figure 5.1). During exercise, the muscles become engorged with blood, and the pressure within the anterior compartment increases and stretches the fascia to the point of causing pain. When exercise is stopped (often because of the pain), the blood leaves the muscles, and the pressure in the anterior compartment is relieved.

This phenomenon, *compartment syndrome*, is most common in competitive athletes, among whom it is a common overuse injury. In recreational exercisers, however, compartment syndrome may occur when the pace or length of exercise is increased too rapidly. Also, gradual warmup exercises may prevent the rapid accumulation of blood in the muscles in the compartment. In addition to stretching exercises, heat applied before and after exercise may decrease symptoms. In severe cases in serious

FIGURE 5.1
Anterior compartment syndrome. Hypertrophied muscles are entrapped in the inelastic fascia of the anterior tibia compartment.

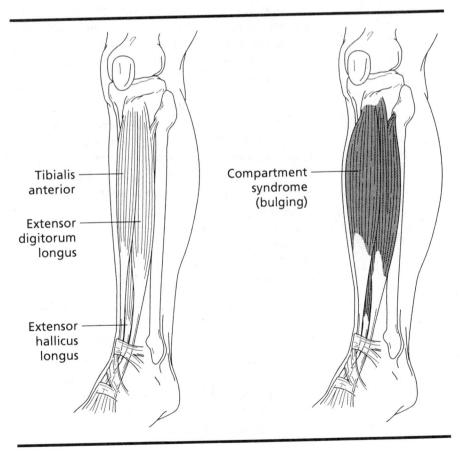

Tibialis anterior

Extensor digitorum longus

Extensor hallicus longus

Compartment syndrome (bulging)

athletes, surgery can be performed to cut the fascia and effectively destroy the constricting compartment. This is a relatively minor procedure, and most athletes undergoing the operation can quickly return to running.

Athletic Injuries

Strains are minor injuries caused by overstretching a muscle or tendon. These injuries can be treated conservatively and usually heal completely in a couple of weeks. Aspirin-like medication is very effective in reducing pain, and immobilization is rarely needed A *sprain* may occur if the over-stretching is severe and the muscle or tendon is torn. Joint sprains were discussed in the previous chapter. A complete tendon or muscle *rupture* is rare, and in this case, only a few (if any) muscle fibers hold the muscle in place. These injuries often need surgical repair, weeks of immobilization and nonuse, and extensive physical rehabilitation to ensure proper healing and return of function.

Shin splints, a common overuse injury in runners, are caused by poor conditioning or warmup and by running on hard, uneven surfaces with improper shoes. The injury causes the muscles in the anterior lower leg to pull away from the bone and also injures tendons in the area. If shin splints occur, ice should be applied for 15 minutes several times a day, and exercise should be stopped until the muscles heal, usually in about three weeks. Proper warmup and an elastic wrap may prevent shin splints from recurring once exercise is resumed.

Other overuse injuries involve either the tendons or ligaments. *Ligament injuries* are common in the knee, especially when lateral movements are forced upon this joint, straining the collateral ligaments. *Tendonitis* (inflammation of the tendon) is common in the elbows, as in "tennis elbow" (affecting the lateral aspect of the joint) or "golfer's elbow" (the medial joint). Tendonitis in the wrist is common in racquetball players and weightlifters. In the treatment of tendonitis, initial immobilization and aspirin-like medications are recommended. If these are not not effective, the area may be injected with local painkillers and cortisone medication. When one returns to the activity that caused the injury, care must be taken to warmup slowly and take frequent breaks during exercise.

Stress fractures are not caused by muscles or ligaments "pulling" on the bone. Rather, they are small disruptions in the bone structure that result from repetitive impact, as in running or jumping. Stress fractures cause an ache in the area of injury that comes on gradually and is made worse by walking or exercising. Often, stress fractures are not detected on regular x-rays, so that a bone scan is needed to make the diagnosis. Because the bone is fractured, immobilization and avoiding the bearing of weight are important for proper healing.

Muscular Dystrophy

Muscular dystrophy is a disease of the muscle fibers. It is not a painful condition, but it does result in profound muscle weakness and may lead to death. The onset of muscle weakness is gradual but typically starts in childhood. Many patienhts are confined to a wheelchair by the age of 12. Despite the weakness, the muscles appear enlarged (hypertrophied), so there is a discrepancy between muscle appearance and function. Muscular dystrophy is a hereditary disease, and one form is transmitted on the X chromosome. Boys with this type of muscular dystrophy rarely live beyond adolescence and usually die of lung infections or choking.

Recent investigations have identified the faulty gene and protein that cause muscular dystrophy. Innovative approaches are being used to try to devise a treatment for muscular dystrophy in which normal genes are injected directly into the muscles so that the proper protein can be produced. Although still experimental, this treatment holds much promise for the future.

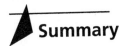

Summary

Muscle injuries are caused by overuse of certain muscles or by traumatic insult. Treatment for muscles injuries involves resting the injured muscle, appropriate use of ice and heat, and aspirin-like medications to reduce pain and inflammation. Full recovery from injuries can be expected, unlike the progressive deterioration in muscle function with muscular dystrophy. New genetic techniques may offer new hope for those suffering from muscular dystrophy.

6 Central Nervous System

CASE PRESENTATION

Mildred was a healthy 57-year-old without significant medical problems. She began noticing a mild headache, which gradually got worse for ten days. The headache occurred in the late afternoon or early evening and felt like a throbbing in her temples. It tended to go away around bedtime and did not wake her up at night. She felt well otherwise and had a normal appetite.

She saw her doctor because she was worried that she had a brain tumor. She was taking no medications except estrogen for menopausal symptoms. Her physical exam, including a detailed evaluation of neurological function, was entirely normal. When further questioned, Mildred admitted being under increased stress recently because her daughter was getting married the following month and she had been busy with the preparations.

Her physician told Mildred that she was suffering from tension headaches and that a CAT scan to look for a brain tumor wasn't needed. She started taking medication for her headaches and enrolled in a stress reduction class. Her headaches soon resolved, and she was able to enjoy her daughter's wedding.

Questions

1. What are tension headaches?
2. Why do some brain tumors cause headaches?
3. Why is a neurological evaluation important?
4. What are migraine headaches?

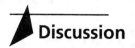

Discussion

Neurology is the study of disorders and diseases of the nervous system. A *neurologist* is a physician specializing in the diagnosis and treatment of these diseases. A *neurosurgeon* is a surgeon who operates on the brain, spinal cord, peripheral and central nerves, and vertebral column.

Special radiological studies are available to assist in the diagnosis of central nervous system disorders. A *CAT scan (computerized axial tomography)* is a special x-ray that displays the brain and vertebral column in horizontal slices. It is used to detect tumors, strokes, and bleeding. An *MRI (magnetic resonance imaging)* is similar to a CAT scan but provides higher resolution of brain structures. A *PET scan (positron emission tomography)* gives information about the blood supply to the brain and metabolic activity.

Two other useful tests are an *EEG (electroencephalogram)* and a *lumbar puncture*. An EEG is a recording of the brain's electrical activity. It is useful in the diagnosis of seizures, and impaired function. A lumbar puncture (spinal tap) is used to sample and study the cerebrospinal fluid. It is especially helpful in diagnosing an infection or bleeding.

Spinal cord injuries are caused by trauma to the vertebral column as in automobile or motorcycle accidents or diving injuries (usually in shallow water). If permanent damage is done, the amount of dysfunction depends on the level at which the spinal cord is injured. For example, *paraplegia* connotes the paralysis of two extremities, usually the legs. *Quadriplegia* means that all four extremities are paralyzed and the level of injury to the spinal cord is higher. Neck injuries that disrupt neuronal activity to the diaphragm cause death. The residual function following a spinal cord injury can be influenced in some instances by rehabilitation, so that optimal usage of the extremities can be obtained.

Headaches

Most people suffer from a headache at some time in their lives, and many are plagued with recurrent headaches requiring some form of treatment. For many people, a certain level of fear is associated with a headache, because the thought of a brain tumor comes to mind. It is true that brain tumors cause headaches, but these tumors are rare, and most headaches are the more common migraine or tension variety. Infection and intracranial bleeding can also cause headaches (Figure 6.1).

Tension headaches are the most common, accounting for 80% of all headaches. They are caused by contraction of the muscles in the neck and scalp. These contractions are typically brought on by emotional or mental stress. Another very common cause of tension headaches is depression, and in this setting, treating the depression may alleviate the headache symptoms. Tension headaches are described as a band-like tightness or pressure, which is most often bilateral. Sometimes the pain can be throbbing, sharp, or localized to a certain area. Many treatment options are available, including stress reduction, biofeedback, massage, and analgesic medications.

Migraine headaches affect 5% to 10% of all headache sufferers. They were thought to be caused by vascular abnormalities. However, it now appears that a complex interaction of hormones, neurotransmitters, and vessel tone contributes to migraine headaches. These headaches are often preceded by an aura of visual, auditory, olfactory, or peripheral sensations. Dizziness, confusion, hallucinations, and even partial paralaysis can also occur. The throbbing migraine headache that follows can be totally debilitating. Several medical treatments can be quite effective in alleviating the symptoms of these headaches.

When a brain tumor is present, the pressure of the tumor and swelling around it can cause a headache (see Figure 6.1). One unique feature of this type of headache is that the neuronal area adjacent to the tumor will also be affected, resulting in local dysfunction of the nervous system in addition to the headache. For example, weakness in one limb, slurred speech, or visual changes may accompany the headache. Subtle impairment of the CNS may persist after the headache and can usually be detected by a physical examination. Headaches due to brain tumors are often continuous, localized to the involved area, occur during sleep, and cause nausea, vomiting, and lack of appetite. A CAT scan is useful in diagnosing a brain tumor.

Seizures

Seizures are the result of disorganized electrical brain discharges. These are manifested by uncontrollable, random, sporadic activity that can be motor, sensory, or mental. Seizures affect 1% of the population and are common among children and young adults. The symptoms of a seizure vary greatly, from generalized, body twitching and jerking to lapses of consciousness, to focal loss of motor control. The symptoms are determined by the area of the brain where the "electrical storm" first arises. All seizures have a sudden onset and a definite ending point, but the length of a seizure may vary from seconds to hours.

The diagnosis of a seizure disorder can be very difficult at times because the periods between seizures are completely normal. The physical exam is normal as well and the diagnostic study for seizures, the electroencephalogram, or EEG, is often normal. During a seizure the EEG is abnormal, showing characteristic electrical spikes. Sometimes, this electrical activity can be elicited with sensory stimulation or sleep deprivation. Rarely, a CAT scan reveals a tumor, mass, stroke, or some other structural cause of the seizure.

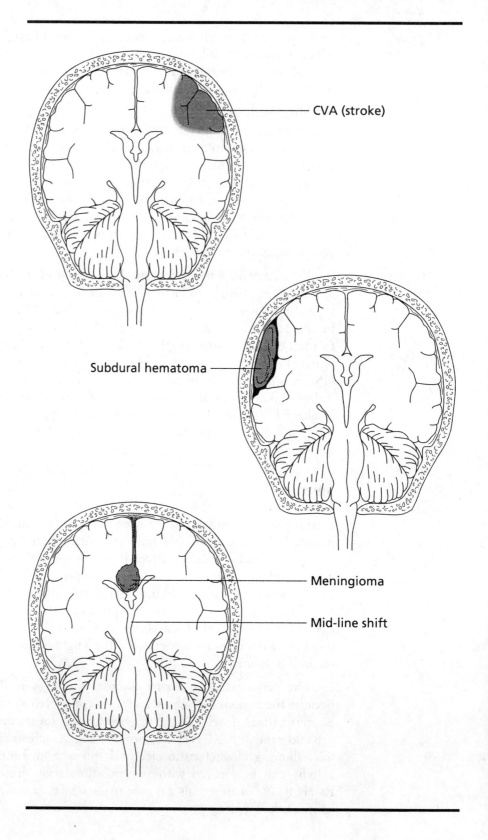

CVA (stroke)

Subdural hematoma

Meningioma

Mid-line shift

There are several specific causes of seizure activity, but most cases of *epilepsy* (repeated seizure activity) have no clear etiology. Infections, drug and alcohol withdrawal, head injuries, strokes, and cancers can cause seizure activity. Once the underlying cause of the seizure is corrected or treated, the seizures do not recur. Persons with epilepsy, on the other hand, often have repeated seizures. After the first seizure occurs, there is a 30% chance of another one within three years. When the second seizure occurs, a person is considered to have epilepsy if no other cause of the seizures is found. Without medical treatment, only 10% to 30% of these persons will not suffer from repeated seizures, but with therapy, the remission rate is much higher (almost 80%).

Treatment of seizures depends largely on the seizure type. Medications are generally effective but carry many side effects, and close follow-up and blood tests are required. New surgical techniques, which isolate the area of seizure activity in the brain, are being used for persons who don't respond to medications. Those afflicted face some limitations on activities that would be dangerous if a seizure occurred (flying, rock climbing), and careful consideration should be given to seizure control before driving a car. Pregnancy carries a higher risk for women who have seizures, and birth defects are more common. Despite these caveats, persons with seizures can engage in normal activities and can seek full, productive employment.

Brain Tumors

Brain tumors are either primary tumors arising from neuronal tissues or metastatic tumors from a cancer elsewhere in the body. Both cause symptoms when they reach a certain size and cause compression on the nervous tissue or impair the flow of blood or cerebrospinal fluid. The most common symptoms include headache (unrelenting, often at night), seizures, decreased mental status, or focal neurological deficits of sensory or motor function. On physical examination, these defects are evident and diagnosis is confirmed with a CAT scan or MRI.

Primary brain tumors affect persons of all ages, including children (see Figure 6.1). Typically, the tumors are removed at time of biopsy unless their location would make surgical removal life threatening or result in permanent disability. It is important to obtain a biopsy of primary brain tumors because different tumor types respond to different types of treatment. Most will shrink with radiation therapy, but the total amount of radiation

---

FIGURE 6.1
Demonstration of central nervous system disorders. A stroke is demonstrated as inadequate blood supply caused by an embolus or thrombus. A subdural hematoma, or bleeding into the subdural space, causes headache. Meningioma is a primary CNS tumor. The mass causes a shift in the ventral midline, resulting in symptoms.

that the brain can tolerate is limited. Chemotherapy is effective in some cancers. An individual with a malignant brain tumor generally survives between two and five years, with fewer than 20% of patients living more than five years.

Stroke

A *stroke* is called a *cerebral vascular accident* (CVA). A CVA is a neurological event caused by inadequate blood supply to an area of the brain. This serious disease takes a huge medical and social toll. The survival rate from a CVA is only 50% to 80% at one month. Many patients will no longer be able to live independently and will require assistance to carry out daily activities or even admission into a nursing home. In addition, persons are more susceptible to other diseases following a stroke.

The symptoms of a stroke depend on the specific CNS area affected and include loss of coordination, motor loss, sensory deficits, speech abnormalities, and changes in mental status. Symptoms have a sudden onset and may progress rapidly. They may last only seconds to a few minutes, or the neurological deficit may be permanent. Neurological deficits may completely resolve in three weeks. Improvement in function can continue beyond that time, but return to completely normal function is less likely.

There are three causes of CVAs. First, bleeding into the CNS parenchyma or dura mater impairs CNS function. Treatment for CNS bleeding is surgical evacuation of the blood when possible. Second, clot formation at a site of vessel narrowing caused by a cholesterol plaque compromises blood flow and may interrupt it altogether. This clot formation is called a *thrombus*. If blood supply is absent for a few hours, the CNS tissue dies and permanent neurological damage occurs. Third, a blood clot formed in the heart or the carotid arteries may break loose and be carried with the blood until it becomes lodged in a smaller cerebral vessel. Here the *embolus* blocks blood flow to the area supplied by the vessel (see Figure 6.1).

The diagnosis of a CVA is based on the clinical history and on findings of neurological impairment in a physical exam. A CAT scan performed at the onset of symptoms will reveal only evidence of bleeding. Usually, it takes 24 to 48 hours before a stroke can be detected by a CAT scan. Then, the location and size of the CVA can be determined.

The treatment of a CVA depends largely on the underlying cause. If bleeding is present, surgical correction of the bleeding or evacuation of blood from the skull may be helpful. If a thrombus or embolus is suspected, medications that prevent clot formation may be used. Rehabilitation is very important and should be started as soon as the person is medically stable. If cholesterol plaque in the carotid arteries is the culprit, surgery can be performed to bypass the area of blockage thus providing an alternate route for blood to reach the brain.

There are several risk factors for developing a CVA. High blood pressure is a major risk factor, and its treatment probably accounts for a decrease in the number of strokes in the United States in recent years. Heart disease and cigarette smoking also contribute to the risk for stroke. Persons who have "minor strokes" in which symptoms last seconds to minutes are at especially high risk of a more devastating CVA. These symptoms should be reported to a physician immediately so that appropriate evaluation and treatment can be initiated.

Dementia

Dementia is a disease affecting millions of elderly persons. It is defined as the progressive deterioration of mental and cognitive function. The onset of symptoms is usually gradual over the course of months or years and may progress rapidly or slowly. Memory loss, confusion, and changes in behavior and personality are the hallmark symptoms of dementia. Symptoms are not always apparent to persons with dementia, and excuses and rationalization for their behavior are common. Symptoms may progress to a point at which those afflicted no longer recognize family members and lose daily functioning.

There are several types of dementia with specific causes. Cerebral degeneration is common, but a clear cause of this disease is not known. Alzheimer's disease appears to have a genetic cause, and characteristic changes in the brain tissue are present. Persons with AIDS often have dementia, possibly due to CNS infection with HIV. Persons that have suffered from multiple strokes (usually small ones caused by high blood pressure) often have dementia. Dementia may accompany severe depression, brain tumors, trauma to the head, alcoholism, and other disorders.

Treatment of dementia is supportive care and attention. Rarely, the underlying cause can be corrected (depression, tumors, other diseases). Many persons require constant supervision and care, which a family cannot realistically provide. When the disease reaches this point, nursing home care or other long-term medical facilities may best meet the needs of both the patient and the family.

Parkinson's Disease

Parkinson's disease is very common, affecting 1% of those over age 65. This disease can markedly alter lifestyle, as severe impairment in motor control occurs. The four hallmark features of Parkinson's disease are 1) a fine tremor that is present at rest but becomes worse with intentional movements such as eating or writing, 2) muscle rigidity exhibited as stiffness, 3) a generalized slowing of motion, and 4) a loss of postural tone and reflexes. These symptoms are usually progressive and are marked by slow speech, drooling, a wide, unsteady gait, and tremor.

A review of brain structure and function allows one to predict that the region of the brain involved in Parkinson's disease is one involved in the control of movement. The underlying problem is located in the basal ganglia. In Parkinson's disease, a lack of the neurotransmitter *dopamine* in the basal ganglia produces the abnormalities of movement. Because dopamine cannot permeate the blood-brain barrier, administering it as a medication is not effective in treating the disease. Therefore, two options are to give the precursor molecule needed for dopamine synthesis, L-dopa, or to give bromocriptine, a compound that binds to dopamine receptors; both of these can cross the blood-brain barrier. These treatments achieve variable results. Recent research has been directed toward implanting neural tissue, sometimes fetal in origin, into the region of the brain containing the basal ganglia. The transplanted tissue is chosen because it is capable of producing dopamine. Maybe a precursor of "brain transplantation" will become an option for patients with Parkinson's disease!

Multiple Sclerosis

Multiple sclerosis is a disease caused by destruction of the myelin sheaths that encase neurons. When myelin is destroyed, the conduction properties of neurons are impaired, and information cannot be transmitted. The destruction of the myelin occurs randomly and sporadically. This results in episodes of neurologic dysfunction, which can attack cranial, motor, sensory, and autonomic neurons. The most common symptoms involve vision (double vision, temporary blindness) and motor function (weakness, paralysis, lack of coordination). Sensory dysfunction (numbness, tingling) and autonomic imbalance (lack of control of bowel and bladder) are also apparent. Symptoms flare intermittently and may last for minutes or be permanent. Most of the time these episodes resolve with time and medical treatment, but the disease is progressive and can lead to death.

Meningitis

Meningitis is an infection of the meninges and cerebrospinal fluid. Although it is potentially fatal, if the cause is bacterial, it is curable with prompt antibiotic therapy. The symptoms include fever, stiff neck and headache. Nausea, vomiting, light sensitivity, and hearing deficits may also occur. The physical exam is very helpful. Avoiding light, inability to touch the chin to the chest, and a rigid neck all point to the diagnosis. Blood tests reveal an elevated white blood cell count. The diagnosis is confirmed with a lumbar puncture and analysis of the cerebrospinal fluid. The spinal fluid pressure is elevated, and the fluid contains white blood cells and bacteria. Bacterial meningitis can progress rapidly, and antibiotic therapy is essential. Viral meningitis is less serious and usually does not even require hospitalization or medications. Various fungi can cause meningitis as well and require very aggressive treatment.

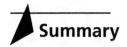

Summary

Diseases of the CNS can be devastating because one's mental function and sense of well-being are affected. These illnesses offer a diagnostic challenge, but too often the treatment options are limited, and symptoms persist. Strokes and dementia are prevalent diseases that consume huge amounts of medical, social, and economic resources. Because cognitive and emotional functions are jeopardized, these diseases are particularly trying to family members, and long-term care is often burdensome.

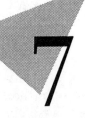

7 Peripheral Nervous System

CASE PRESENTATION

Jane, 25 years old, worked as a secretary for a business. After several months of having her hands "fall asleep" during the night, she began getting up because of the pain and trying to massage her hands to decrease the throbbing. She did not have symptoms during the day and felt well otherwise. One night while she was up, she had difficulty opening a bottle of soda, and the next morning she made an appointment to see her doctor.

On physical exam, her hands were warm and had good pulses and color. Her hand strength was normal, and reflexes were intact. She had normal sensory detection to temperature, proprioception, and pinprick. The doctor asked Jane to forcefully hyperextend her wrist and maintain that position. Within a few minutes, her symptoms were present. When rechecked, the sensation to pinprick was diminished in some of her fingers.

Jane was told she had carpal tunnel syndrome. Medication, special tests, and physical therapy were recommended. In retrospect, she recalled that about a year before, she had started working heavily on a new computer at work.

Questions

1. What is carpal tunnel syndrome?
2. What causes it?
3. What other disorders affect the peripheral nervous system?

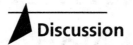

Discussion

Diseases of the peripheral nervous system affect the somatic and autonomic systems. Neurologists and neurosurgeons have expertise in these disorders as well as in disorders of the CNS. In addition to the x-ray studies described in the previous chapter, two studies that assist in the diagnosis of peripheral nervous system diseases. An *EMG* (*electromyogram*) measures the electrical activity of a muscle, and *nerve conduction studies* measure the time of conduction down a nerve. Checking reflexes, motor strength, and sensory perception all aid in localizing the disorder.

Carpal Tunnel Syndrome

Carpal tunnel syndrome can be a very debilitating disease and is responsible for a significant amount of missed work. Carpal tunnel syndrome is the entrapment of the median nerve in the carpal tunnel in the wrist. The carpal tunnel is formed by the bones in the wrist and the transverse carpal ligament. In addition to the median nerve, nine muscle tendons to the hand also pass through the carpal tunnel en route to the hand. Any condition that "crowds," or impinges on, the median nerve can cause symptoms of carpal tunnel syndrome. This is most frequently a tendonitis causing a swelling around the median nerve.

At the onset, symptoms typically occur at night, with resolution of symptoms during the day. Numbness and tingling in the hands gradually develop and may progress to symptoms of burning, aching, pain, and incoordination. There may be a dull pain through the arm and excessive sweating in the hand. Symptoms usually go away with rubbing, shaking, or dangling the hands. Eventually, the symptoms occur in the day and inhibit work performance and household tasks.

In early stages of the disease, the physical exam is normal. Occasionally, symptoms can be elicited by hyperextending or flexing the wrist or by tapping on the carpal tunnel. At later stages, decreased sensation in the lateral three digits, lateral half of the fourth digit, and thenar eminence develops followed by decreased strength in these areas (Figure 7.1). Diagnosis is confirmed with nerve conduction studies, which are usually positive even when the exam is normal.

Workers who perform repeated tasks with their hands are at greatest risk for developing carpal tunnel syndrome. These include typists, food processors, packers, painters, carpenters, and many others. These people develop a tendonitis which leads to carpal tunnel syndrome. This syndrome is also common in pregnant women (fluid retention and swelling), in persons with rheumatoid arthritis (joint inflammation encroachment), in diabetics (nerve swelling), and with other structural abnormalities that impinge on the median nerve in the carpal tunnel.

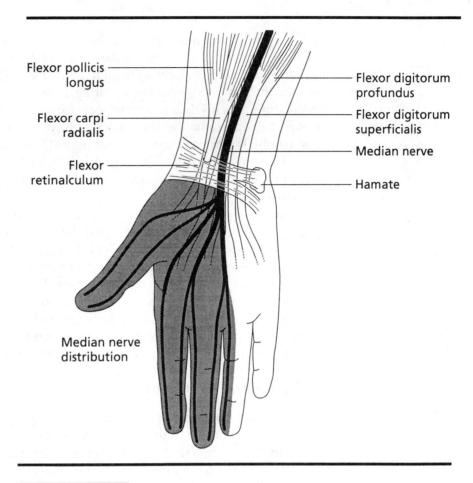

Flexor pollicis longus

Flexor carpi radialis

Flexor retinalculum

Flexor digitorum profundus

Flexor digitorum superficialis

Median nerve

Hamate

Median nerve distribution

FIGURE 7.1

Carpal tunnel syndrome. The median nerve is trapped in the carpal tunnel and causes symptoms in the distribution of this nerve.

Treatment of carpal tunnel syndrome is multifactorial. Splints that immobilize the wrist in the neutral position can be worn at night and at rest. These are very effective at relieving annoying symptoms. Oral medications and local steroid injections, which relieve pain and decrease inflammation, offer temporary help, although symptoms often recur once treatment is stopped. Surgery to "release" the median nerve is reserved for persons with refractory symptoms. Usually the results are good. Occupational and physical therapy should be prescribed to prevent further injury at the workplace and to guide rehabilitation.

Tetanus And Shingles

Tetanus and shingles are two diseases dependent on transport via the peripheral nerves. *Tetanus* is caused by a bacterium that is common in the soil. When this organism enters the body via a wound, it releases a toxin (poison). The toxin travels to the spinal cord through the motor axon and is transmitted to the inhibitory neurons. The toxin blocks neurotransmission in the inhibitory neurons, resulting in increased and uncontrolled motor tone. Tetany is a sustained contraction in the affected muscle groups. Lockjaw (tetany of the masseter muscle) is common, but generalized painful tetany can occur and lead to death by compromising ventilation. These symptoms may be triggered by a variety of factors. Tetanus infection is treated by a combination of therapies and is prevented by immunization.

Shingles is caused by the herpes zoster virus. Once a herpes infection occurs, most frequently as chicken pox, the virus can remain dormant in the ganglia indefinitely. When the body is under stress (disease, anxiety), the virus seizes the opportunity to travel down the sensory axon and causes infection along the course of the nerve root. The lesions are painful, red blisters that usually occur in a streak on the skin along a dermatone and do not cross the midline of the body. Diagnosis is largely clinical, and treatment involves topical ointments and pain control, although new research is under way into the use of acyclovir, an antiviral agent.

Guillain-Barré Syndrome

Guillain-Barré syndrome is caused by demyelination of neuronal axons. Symptoms appear one to three weeks following a viral illness. Progressive loss of motor function starts in the lower extremities and ascends to involve the upper extremities and even the cranial nerves. If the respiratory muscles are affected, a ventilation machine is needed to support breathing. The muscle weakness may be accompanied by pain in the posterior regions of the legs, but the sensory nerves are left intact. The autonomic nervous system can be affected, altering blood pressure, body temperature, and heart rhythms. Death occurs in fewer than 5% of individuals with Guillain-Barré syndrome, but hospitalization for support during the illness is necessary in most instances. Approximately 80% will reach a nearly total recovery, but it may take many months.

Local Pain Control

Pain control is an important aspect of medical practice. Local anesthetics (painkillers) are used widely to treat or prevent pain. These medications often work by inhibiting the flow of sodium ions into cells, thereby blocking the production of action potentials. *Novocaine* and *Xylocaine* are two familiar anesthetics that work in this manner and cause a numb, painless state in the areas where they are administered. Nerves in the area of anesthetic administration are blocked to varying degrees depending on size. For example, certain small autonomic fibers and certain sensory fibers are affected long before the large, myelinated fibers of motor neurons. This allows adequate pain control to be achieved without the loss of motor function, an important component of local anesthesia.

The forms of local pain control include topical anesthesia, local anesthesia, nerve block, and spinal anesthesia. Topical anesthesia refers to the application of the agent to the surface to be anesthetized. The effectiveness of a topical agent relies on its ability to penetrate a surface such as the skin (as in the treatment of burns and itching), the eye (as in the treatment of eye infections or injuries), or mucus linings (as in treating the mouth, throat, and vagina). The anesthetic diffuses into the area to which it is applied and blocks nerve conduction in this location. Most anesthetics cannot penetrate all the way through intact, undamaged skin; thus, topical applications are not effective for treating pain that is deep to the skin, such as that in muscles or joints.

Local anesthesia is achieved by injecting the medication into a specific area. This technique is used commonly in dental work, suturing of wounds, and minor surgeries. The duration of the pain relief depends on the amount and type of medication injected, and the injection may be repeated during the procedure to ensure adequate pain control. The size of the area that can be anesthetized with this technique is usually small.

Peripheral nerve block is an extremely effective method for achieving pain control over a larger, deeper area. Instead of numbing the area directly, the anesthetist injects a substance in the area of the nerve or ganglion supplying the area. For example, the entire finger can be anesthetized by injecting medication into the lateral and medial sides of the finger at the base, thus blocking all sensory innervation. Ganglionic blocks can be achieved in the same way, are effective over large areas, and are particularly useful in the treatment of pain associated with cancer.

Spinal anesthesia is often used in place of general anesthesia if surgery is localized to the lower extremity. For example, this technique may be used in orthopedic, urological, or dermatological procedures. The medication is injected into the vertebral cavity in the subdural space and blocks all of the nerves leaving the portion of the spinal cord that is bathed in the anesthetic. Unfortunately, the autonomic and somatic motor nerves are blocked by this procedure as well, and a drop in blood pressure due to autonomic interference can be dangerous.

Caffeine

Caffeine is a drug in extremely common use. More than 30 million pounds of coffee is consumed yearly in the United States alone, amounting to a daily average of about two cups per person. Caffeine is a naturally occurring substance and is found in coffee beans, cocoa beans, cola nuts, tea, and other materials. It is consumed both for its flavor and for the physiological and psychological effects it produces.

Caffeine both stimulates the CNS and activates the PNS. It acts by blocking the degradation of cyclic AMP (see Chapter 14). Cyclic AMP, a so-called "second messenger," is formed by the binding of certain chemical signals to adrenergic receptors. In the presence of caffeine, more cyclic AMP is available, and it is available for a longer period. Centrally, this effect causes the stimulation of the cerebral cortex and produces a heightened state of awareness, reduced fatigue, and, paradoxically, a sense of relaxation. Peripherally, caffeine constricts most blood vessels (which can elevate blood pressure), increases sweating, increases intestinal motility, increases urination, causes stronger and faster heart contractions, and increases metabolic rate. Basically, caffeine produces influences similar to those of generalized sympathetic activation.

The four most common sources of caffeine in the diets of most people are coffee, tea, colas, and chocolate. The amount of caffeine in these substances varies greatly. For example, a 5-ounce cup of drip coffee contains 150 mg of caffeine, a cup of instant coffee about 50 mg, and a cup of decaffeinated coffee about 2 mg. A cup of tea brewed for five minutes may contain as much as 50 mg of caffeine; if brewed for one minute it will contain about 30 mg. Colas contain 20 to 50 mg of caffeine per 12-ounce serving. Most herbal teas contain minimal amounts of caffeine. Caffeine is also found in many other food products and in over-the-counter medications for allergies, colds, headaches, dieting, and stimulants to prevent sleep.

The acute side effects of excess caffeine use may include headaches, tremors, diarrhea, anxiety, irritability, hyperactivity, depression, insomnia, and abnormally fast heart rhythms. Dependency on caffeine may also develop if the amount ingested daily exceeds 300 mg. Uneasiness, decreased alertness, and headache are common complaints with caffeine withdrawal. Caffeine may also worsen ulcers in the digestive tract and breast cysts in certain women. The widespread use of this substance has led to its acceptance as a "natural" stimulant, but all casual consumers should consider the possible undesirable effects of caffeine as well as the desirable ones.

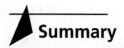

Summary

Disorders of the peripheral nervous system can be localized to a solitary, involved nerve root (carpal tunnel syndrome), or the disease may have a general affect on several peripheral nerves, both somatic and autonomic (Guillain-Barré syndrome). Some neurological diseases affect both the central and peripheral nervous systems (multiple sclerosis), and others are limited to a single nerve root (shingles). A detailed neurological examination, special x-rays, and electrical studies lead to the diagnosis of peripheral nerve disorders. Treatment is determined by the causative agent and severity of the disease.

8 Sensory Organs

CASE PRESENTATIONS

Martha, 14, was at school, her teacher noticed that her right eye was red and sent her to see the school nurse. Martha did not feel sick, had no impairment of her vision on chart testing, and had no fever. She was sent home from school and instructed to see her pediatrician. Later that afternoon, Martha's eye became sore and itchy, and had a yellow discharge. Her pediatrician asked about eye injuries or allergies, and she had had neither. On examination, the conjunctiva of the eye was red and swollen. The iris was spared, and the pupil reacted normally to light stimulation. Again, Martha's vision was normal. The diagnosis of an eye infection was made, and eye drops were prescribed. Martha was instructed to stay home from school until the eye healed, as the infection was highly contagious. Within a few days Martha's eye was normal, and she returned to school.

Martha's grandfather, Jim, was 70 years old and in good health. For two years he had had increasing problems with blurred vision, and he sought medical attention from his ophthalmologist. On physical exam, the corneas of his eyes were opaque. His prescription for glasses was accurate, and a test for glaucoma was negative. The physician told Jim that he had cataracts and recommended surgery. Jim underwent surgery and his vision improved.

Questions

1. How are eye infections different from other diseases of the eye?
2. What are cataracts, and how are they treated?
3. What other disorders cause blindness?
4. What disorders affect other sensory organs, such as the ears?

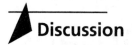 **Discussion**

Vision, hearing, and equilibrium can be affected by diseases, resulting in impairment of senses. Taste and smell are largely spared by disease states. Pain is a sensation that accompanies many diseases and a great deal of medical attention is devoted to relieving pain. Pain treatment must be individualized to suit the severity of the pain, the underlying disease causing the pain, and the specific situation of the person suffering from pain. In fact, there are "pain clinics" that focus only on the treatment of pain.

Optometrists and ophthalmologists specialize in eye disorders. Vision tests are performed routinely to detect myopia (nearsightedness), hyperopia (farsightedness), and astigmatism (uneven focusing) so that glasses or contact lenses can be prescribed. Tests for glaucoma and visualization of the retina should be performed routinely in adults. Otolaryngologists, or ear, nose, and throat doctors, specialize in disorders of these organs. Frequently, hearing disorders are also evaluated by a neurologist. Hearing tests are routinely performed on preschool children to detect hearing loss that may impede learning. Disturbances of equilibrium are common, and most physicians are trained in the diagnosis and treatment of such disorders. Complicated equilibrium disorders are often referred to a neurologist for further evaluation and treatment. For the most part, blood tests and x-ray studies are not useful in the detection of sensory impairments.

Blindness

Several diseases result in blindness. The most common ones are cataracts, glaucoma, and complications of diabetes. Night blindness is an inability to see well in the dark; the rods in the retina do not adequately compensate for diminished light stimulation. Color blindness is the inability to detect certain colors. Persons with red color blindness lack red cones and are unable to detect red light waves. Green color blindness is more common and results from a lack of green cones. Color blindness is more common in males than females due to the hereditary nature of the disorder.

A cataract is the clouding of the lens or capsule of the eye. Cataracts are a common ailment of the elderly, affecting nearly 50% of persons 75 years and older. Cataracts are usually bilateral, but the progression of clouding in each eye may proceed at different rates. Impaired or decreased visual acuity is the predominant symptom of cataracts. The opacity diminishes the amount of light passing through the lens and reaching the retina. Objects can be detected, but there appears to be a fog present. Light halos around objects may also be detected. The process is not painful, and the other components of the eye are not affected. There is no way to predict the progression of cataracts and no treatment to prevent progression. When the vision impairment becomes severe, cataract surgery can be performed. The diseased lens is replaced with an artificial lens which is made of a plastic material. The success rate of surgery is high.

Glaucoma is a disease caused by abnormally high pressure in the anterior cavity of the eye. Elevated pressure is the result of increased production of aqueous humor or decreased removal of it from the anterior chamber. Intraocular pressures increase sufficiently to compress the blood vessels supplying the eye and cause irreversible damage to the retina and optic nerve. The first symptoms are subtle decreases in the field of vision. Objects on the periphery of the visual field are not visualized, a condition called tunnel vision. Loss of peripheral vision may progress to the point of blindness. Blurred vision and seeing a ring of light around objects are also common. Rarely, eye pain, headache, and nausea may be present. Diagnosis is made by measuring the pressure in the anterior chamber by placing an instrument on the eye directly after anesthetizing the eye with drops (Figure 8.1). All persons over the age of 40 should undergo routine screening for glaucoma to detect changes before vision is impaired. Medications can be given to prevent the progression of glaucoma, but once vision

FIGURE 8.1
Glaucoma testing. A tonometer is placed on the anesthetized eye to measure the pressure in the anterior chamber.

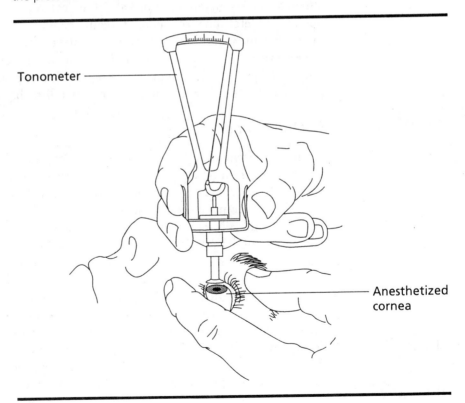

Tonometer

Anesthetized cornea

impairment has occurred, it can not be reversed. Glaucoma accounts for 15% to 20% of blindness in the United States.

Diabetes mellitus will be discussed in the following chapter. Complications of this disease include changes in the nerves and blood vessels, and the eye is particularly prone to damage. Changes in the vascular supply to the eye begin early in the course of diabetes mellitus. As the damage to the vessels progresses, an inadequate blood and oxygen supply to the eye occurs, and small areas of the retina do not function adequately. Gradually, visual acuity is decreased, often to the point of blindness. Persons with diabetes mellitus also suffer from intraocular hemorrhage (bleeding) and from acute retinal detachment, resulting in sudden loss of vision. Surgery is often beneficial in the treatment of these eye diseases, but diabetes remains the leading cause of blindness in the United States.

Conjunctivitis

The most common eye infection is *conjunctivitis*. This is an infection of the conjunctiva and often involves the eyelid as well. The cause is usually a viral or bacterial organism, and both are highly contagious. Infections are spread in the secretions from the eye when an infected person contaminates his or her hands, clothing, or towels. The symptoms of conjunctivitis include mild discomfort, excessive tearing, itching, burning, thick secretions (often yellow), and swelling of the lid. Typically, only one eye is affected, and vision remains normal. A physical exam will confirm the diagnosis and determine the need for emergency treatment if the iris is involved (which rarely occurs). Conjunctivitis is often a self-limited disease (going away without treatment), but topical antibiotics in the form of eye drops will speed recovery in cases of bacterial infections. Healing is complete in days, and there are no residual visual disturbances.

Ear Infections

Ear infections are called *otitis media* (infection of the middle ear) or *otitis externa* (infection of the external canal). Otitis media is very common in children but occurs rarely in adults. The age distribution of this disease is due to the anatomy of the Eustachian tubes, which are nearly horizontal at birth and gradually lengthen to become more vertical. When the tubes are more horizontal, the environment is more conducive for bacteria from the pharynx to enter them and spread to the middle ear. Symptoms include a painful ear, which may itch, swollen, painful lymph nodes; and generalized symptoms of fatigue, fever, and malaise. On examination, the tympanic membrane appears red and bulging from the infected fluid behind it. Treatment is with antibiotics. If recurrent infections occur, hearing may be compromised. In this case, a small plastic tube may be inserted from the external canal across the tympanic membrane to allow the middle ear to drain freely, thus preventing the buildup of infected fluid.

Unlike otitis media, otitis externa is rarely caused by bacteria. Fungal infections are most common, especially when there is water in the external canal. For this reason, otitis externa is referred to as "swimmer's ear" and can be prevented by thorough drying of the ear canal. Local symptoms of itching and pain are present, with or without swollen lymph nodes. The irritation of the external canal can be seen on examination. Treatment is with topical agents administered as ear drops. These same symptoms may occur with excessive buildup of cerumen in the ear canal. This condition is treated by removing the cerumen, sometimes after loosening or moistening the plug with drops. The use of cotton swabs to clean the ears may actually make the situation much worse and should be avoided.

Hearing Loss

The reduction or loss of hearing is called *deafness*. It is a common symptom, affecting over 12 million Americans. In fact, one in five persons over the age of 65 years will have moderate to severe hearing loss. Hearing can be tested in two ways. Auditory tests produce tones of varying intensity (decibels) and tone (frequency). An audiogram plots the decibels and frequencies detected in each ear. Another test involves the use of a vibratory tuning fork. A person can hear the vibration either through the air or via the bone, if the tuning fork is placed on the mastoid process. Tests using a tuning fork help determine which type of hearing loss is present.

There are two types of deafness. In *sensorineural* deafness, the abnormality exists in the cochlea, auditory nerve, or brain. The sound waves are conducted through the middle ear, but the neural processing and transmitting of these impulses are impaired. This type of deafness is common among the elderly. Hearing in the high frequency range is lost first, and friends and family are usually the first to notice the hearing loss. *Conduction deafness* is caused by unsuccessful conduction of sound waves to the cochlea. Defects involving the external canal, tympanic membrane, middle ear, and ossicles result in conduction deafness. Cerumen buildup, tympanic membrane perforation, chronic infections, and ossicular damage cause conduction deafness.

Hearing aids are miniature microphone amplifiers that increase the intensity of sound waves. These devices are particularly effective for sensorineural hearing loss but can also benefit one with conduction deafness. The cost of a hearing aid ranges from $300 to $600.

Dizziness

Dizziness is defined as spatial disorientation or an uncertainness about one's position or motion in relation to the environment. Dizziness is a common symptom. Patients may describe light-headedness, a drunken feeling, fainting, imbalance, or other peculiar feelings. Depending on the cause and severity, actual loss of consciousness may occur. There are numerous causes of dizziness. Hyperventilation is a common cause of chronic dizziness, but more severe problems such as life-threatening heart rhythms or early strokes may also cause dizziness. Dehydration, medications, some neurological diseases, and inner ear disorders are common culprits.

Vertigo is a sensation of the external environment spinning or turning. For example, this sensation is experienced after getting off a merry-go-round. It is caused by a problem with the inner ear labyrinth or cranial nerve. Vertigo is generally considered a symptom distinct from dizziness. The most common version is positional vertigo, in which symptoms occur when the head is turned or moved quickly. Symptoms are usually self-limited, last weeks to months, and may recur years later.

Ménière's syndrome is a constellation of symptoms consisting of vertigo, hearing loss, and a ringing in the ears (tinnitis). It is caused by excess fluid and pressure in the cochlea and the labyrinth. Medical and surgical treatments are available for those who suffer from Ménière's disease.

Motion sickness is caused by vestibular disturbances while moving and affects one-third of the population. Symptoms of vertigo, headache, drowsiness, sweating, nausea, vomiting, and hyperventilation are common. Symptoms usually resolve after a few days on a sea voyage, when one acclimates to the motion. Avoiding activities that provoke symptoms (reading in cars, going below deck on a boat) and focusing on distant objects or the horizon can reduce symptoms. Medications are available for motion sickness and are most effective if taken in anticipation of symptoms instead of when symptoms begin. Most of these medications have side effects, and drowsiness is common.

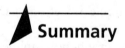

Summary

Disturbances of the eyes and ears result in significant medical problems. Blindness and hearing loss are common, especially in the elderly population. Regular screening for those at risk is an important preventive health measure. Dizziness is a common symptom among all age groups and is frequently attributed to an imbalance of equilibrium. Infection of the outer canal and middle ear, as well as conjunctivitis, occur with great frequency in children and less commonly in adults. Pain control is an important part of medicine, and new medications and treatment modalities are constantly being developed to relieve pain.

9 Endocrine System

CASE PRESENTATIONS

Sally, 11 years old, had had a normal childhood and had been a bright and active youngster. For a couple of months, however, Sally had had less energy to keep up with her friends. She was feeling more fatigued and was performing less well in school. Her parents also noted a significant weight loss, though her appetite increased. She was also urinating quite frequently and was drinking excessive amounts of water. Her parents made an appointment for her to see her family physician.

On physical examination, Sally appeared very thin and dehydrated. Her breath had a peculiar odor of acetone. Otherwise, there were no abnormal findings. The physician suspected diabetes mellitus and ordered a urine sample and blood test to confirm his diagnosis. Sally and her parents were told that she did have diabetes mellitus and that she would need to take insulin shots for the rest of her life.

Mr. Mackey was Sally's next door neighbor. He was 71 years old and enjoyed his retirement by relaxing at home and reading. He had had no health-related complaints and went for a routine physical with his doctor. On physical exam, he was moderately overweight and had borderline high blood pressure. A blood test was obtained to check his cholesterol and glucose. Both were elevated, and the glucose level was so high that it was checked again. Mr. Mackey was told that he had diabetes mellitus and was instructed to loose weight, exercise regularly, and change his diet. Six months later, his glucose level was much better, and he did not have to start taking oral medications for his diabetes mellitus.

Questions

1. What is diabetes mellitus?
2. Why are the two case presentations so different in symptoms and treatment?
3. What causes diabetes mellitus?
4. What other diseases can be caused by endocrine disorders?

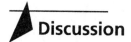

Discussion

Endocrinology is the study of the endocrine system and the diseases that affect this system. An *endocrinologist* is a physician specializing in endocrinology. Most of these disorders are caused by over- or under-production of a specific hormone or by the body's ability to respond to a given amount of hormone. Therefore, measurement of the concentration of hormones in the blood is a very useful diagnostic tool. In addition to the actual hormone level, other metabolic substances that are influenced by hormones can be measured. For example, in one form of diabetes mellitus the primary abnormality is insufficient production of insulin. Without insulin, the glucose in the blood cannot be taken into the cells, and the blood glucose level is abnormally elevated. It is easier and more accurate to measure the glucose in the blood than to measure the actual amount of insulin. Specialized scans utilizing radioactive tracers are also helpful in the diagnosis of endocrine disorders, especially of the thyroid gland.

Thyroid Disease

Thyroid diseases are very common disorders of the endocrine system. Either overproduction or inadequate production of thyroid hormone causes symptoms and requires medical treatment. When excessive thyroid hormone is produced, *hyperthyroidism* occurs. *Hypothyroidism* is the condition in which inadequate amounts of thyroid hormone are produced. *Goiter* is a term to describe an enlarged thyroid gland. It can be totally benign (asymptomatic) or may be associated with hyper- or hypothyroidism. Likewise, a *thyroid nodule* (a localized enlargement of thyroid tissue within the gland) can be benign or associated with thyroid disease.

Blood tests and thyroid scans are useful tools in the diagnosis and treatment of thyroid disorders. The level of thyroid hormones (T3, T4, and total thyroid hormone) can be measured in the blood. Thyroid-stimulating hormone (TSH) can also be measured. These measurements permit the diagnosis of hyper- or hypothyroidism. Certain autoantibodies (antibodies made by the body that attack its own tissues) can be detected in the blood to determine the cause of the thyroid disorder. These measurements of hormones can not only assist in diagnosis but can also determine the effects of treatment. Thyroid scans show the activity of the thyroid gland or nodule by detecting the uptake of radioactively labeled iodine. Finally, a thyroid biopsy may be necessary to confirm a diagnosis.

Hyperthyroidism has many causes. The most common cause is *Grave's disease*, which is an autoimmune disorder. It is caused by the production of autoantibodies that stimulate the thyroid gland to produce excessive amounts of thyroid hormone. The overproduction of thyroid hormone leads to symptoms of nervousness, pounding heart, weight loss, goiter, heat intolerance, weakness, shortness of breath, and protruding eyes. The eye changes are probably antibody mediated. Diagnosis of hyperthyroidism is made by blood tests, which reveal high levels of thyroid hormone and low levels of TSH. Sometimes, antibodies can also be detected. The treatment of hyperthyroidism is directed at eliminating excess thyroid hormone or prevention of hormone production. Medications are effective in some persons. Others require treatment to destroy the thyroid gland with radioactivity or surgical removal of the gland. Once this is accomplished, thyroid replacement medication is needed to prevent hypothyroidism.

Hypothyroidism can also be caused by autoantibodies, as in *Hashimoto's thyroiditis*. The destruction of the thyroid gland results in inadequate thyroid hormone production. Also, diseases of the pituitary gland in which TSH is underproduced cause hypothyroidism. The symptoms of hypothyroidism include fatigue, intolerance to cold, muscle stiffness and aches, constipation, depression, hair loss, and dry skin. These symptoms come on very gradually and may not be readily detected by the affected individual. Thyroid hormone measured in the blood is decreased in hypothyroidism, and the TSH may be elevated (primary thyroid gland abnormality) or depressed (inadequate TSH production by the pituitary gland). In either case, treatment is with thyroid replacement in the form of an oral medication taken once a day.

Diabetes Mellitus

Diabetes mellitus is a disease characterized by the inability of cells to utilize glucose and by elevated blood glucose levels. In a sense, "starvation" occurs in an environment of excess glucose, because insulin production is inadequate or the cells cannot respond to insulin that is present. There are two clinically distinct types of diabetes.

Type I diabetes mellitus is caused by inadequate production of insulin by the beta cells in the pancreas. It is an autoimmune disease in which autoantibodies attack and destroy the beta cells. Type I diabetes mellitus typically occurs in childhood, but can affect adults as well. The symptoms come on gradually and include weight loss in the face of an increased appetite, excessive drinking and urination, and weakness. This leads to dehydration, and excessive acid production from fat metabolism can be life threatening. Diagnosis is confirmed by detecting glucose and acids in the urine, and blood tests reveal elevated glucose levels, possibly ten times normal. Treatment of Type I diabetes mellitus is by insulin replacement. Unfortunately, insulin cannot be taken orally, and daily (or multiple) injections are required. Recent advances have led to the development of an insulin pump, which continuously delivers insulin to the body.

Type II diabetes mellitus is more common than Type I and accounts for 80% to 90% of diabetic persons. The underlying abnormality in Type II diabetes mellitus is that cells are not responsive to the insulin in the blood, a condition called insulin resistance. The symptoms are minimal, and many persons are asymptomatic. Type II diabetes mellitus is often diagnosed in asymptomatic people by routine blood work or screening. The first line of treatment is weight loss, diet modifications, and exercise, which will improve the body's sensitivity to insulin. Oral medications that improve insulin secretion or responsiveness may be effective if these measures are not. In some instances, insulin injections are required to overcome insulin resistance.

The complications of diabetes mellitus are the same regardless of the type (Figure 9.1). Diabetes mellitus is the leading cause of blindness in the United States due to its effects on blood vessels in the eyes. Kidney disease is also common with diabetes mellitus, accounting for most dialysis and transplant patients. Heart attacks and strokes are more common because diabetes mellitus is a risk factor for developing atherosclerosis, or hardening of the arteries. Amputations are necessary at times due to inadequate blood supply to an extremity or because a sore cannot heal properly. Peripheral nerves are also affected, resulting in impaired sensory function. These complications are devastating, and there is a great need for more research to prevent diabetes-related illnesses.

Pituitary Tumors

The most common tumors originating in the brain are in the pituitary gland. In over half of these tumors, the clinical evidence for an endocrine abnormality is oversecretion of a pituitary hormone. The majority of these abnormalities are prolactin-producing tumors called *prolactinomas*. The so-called "nonfunctioning" tumors are the second most common type of pituitary tumor. They do not oversecrete a functional hormone. It is interesting that nearly 10% of the nonfunctioning tumors are composed of cells that do, in fact, contain hormones. How could a tumor composed of hormone-containing cells not result in the oversecretion of a functional hormone? The answer is that the cells of these tumors produce an abnormal hormone that is incapable of exerting a biological affect on target organs. (Recall that a hormone's structure is crucial for its proper function. Any abnormality in the synthesis of a hormone may alter its structure.) Tumors producing adrenocorticotropic hormone and growth hormone releasing

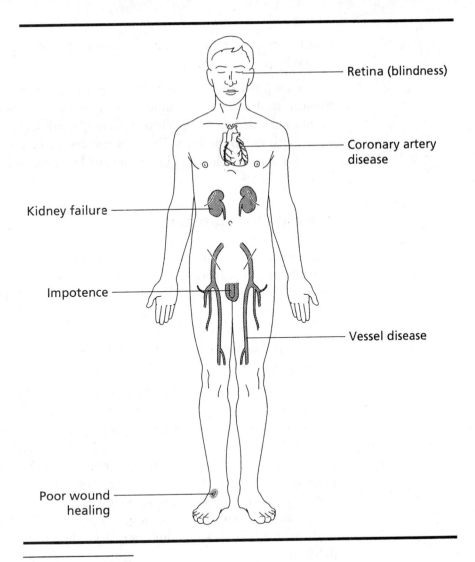

F I G U R E   9 . 1
Diabetes affects the blood vessels and nervous tissue, resulting in widespread complications.

hormone are infrequent. Tumors producing thyroid-stimulating hormone, luteinizing hormone, and follicle-stimulating hormone are quite rare.

Prolactinomas are particularly symptomatic in females because they cause menstrual irregularities, infertility, and lactation. Males with these tumors come to medical attention for infertility and sexual dysfunction less frequently than women, but prolactinomas occur with about equal frequency in the two sexes. A unique feature of prolactinomas is that they can be treated with medication that mimics the actions of the neurotransmitter dopamine, because dopamine inhibits the release of prolactin. It is worth noting that many cases of increased prolactin secretion are not caused by pituitary tumors.

Other problems that arise with pituitary tumors are related to the anatomical location of these tumors. For example, headaches may develop. Additionally, deficits in the visual field may result if the tumor impairs the visual pathway to the brain. Pituitary tumors are diagnosed by testing the blood for abnormal levels of hormones and by examining a CAT scan of the head.

Adrenal Gland Diseases

Diseases of the adrenal gland are not common. *Addison's disease* is caused by inadequate production of cortisol and aldosterone. Symptoms include profound weakness, weight loss, low blood pressure, abdominal pain, nausea, and vomiting. The lack of aldosterone results in salt wasting by the kidneys (in the urine) so that persons crave salt and eat it excessively. Treatment is replacement therapy with glucocorticol and mineralcorticol hormones.

Cushing's disease is caused by excessive levels of cortisol as a result of excessive ACTH production by the pituitary gland. This causes high blood pressure, diabetes, muscle weakness, osteoporosis, and swelling of the face and trunk. Treatment involves halting ACTH production, usually by surgical removal of the pituitary gland. Although Cushing's disease is rare, many persons have Cushing's syndrome. The symptoms are the same, but excess cortisol is the result of treatment with medications for arthritis, lung disease, and many other diseases. Despite the beneficial effects of these "steroid" medications (like prednisone), the side effects can be serious and debilitating.

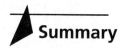

Summary

Diabetes mellitus and thyroid diseases are very common endocrine disorders that affect millions of Americans. Both hypo- and hyperthyroidism can be caused by autoimmune disorders. The symptoms of these two thyroid diseases are opposite due to the effect of thyroid hormone on metabolism. There are two clinical types of diabetes mellitus, with separate causes, symptoms, and treatments. However, the elevated glucose and cellular inability to utilize glucose are common to both types, as are the complications. Other endocrine disorders are uncommon; treatments are directed at supplementing or removing the excess source of hormone.

10 The Heart

CASE PRESENTATION

Mr. Smith, 60, arrived at the emergency room complaining of chest pain. He had been working in his deli that morning when the pain began. It lasted 15 minutes and went away when he stopped working and rested. The pain returned, however, and became unrelenting. He had difficulty breathing, and his wife noted that he had been sweating profusely. She said he had been complaining of "indigestion" off and on for the previous few months.

Mr. Smith was taking a medication for high blood pressure but had no other health problems. His father died of a heart attack at age 54, and his brother just had open heart surgery. He drank five or six beers on the weekends and smoked a pack of cigarettes a day; he used to smoke two packs a day.

On physical exam, Mr. Smith was moderately obese and appeared anxious, short of breath and diaphoretic (sweaty). His blood pressure and pulse were both elevated. There was some fluid in the base of his lungs, his heart had no murmurs, his abdomen was normal, and his feet and hands were cool and clammy.

Immediately, an IV was placed, oxygen was administered, and he was given some nitroglycerine under his tongue. An electrocardiogram (ECG) showed a large heart attack involving the anterior wall of the heart. The physician explained to Mr. Smith that he was having a heart attack and gave him a dose of streptokinase, a drug that dissolves blood clots. Within 30 minutes, Mr. Smith was pain free. He was admitted to the intensive care unit for monitoring and treatment for his myocardial infarction (heart attack).

Questions

1. What is a heart attack?
2. Why are nitroglycerine and oxygen given?
3. What does an ECG show?

4. Why are "clot busters" administered during a heart attack?
5. What is the mortality with a heart attack?
6. Can heart attacks be prevented?

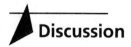

Discussion

Heart disease is the number one killer among American men and women. Nearly 600,000 people die each year of heart disease (especially heart attacks), accounting for one-third of all deaths. Over the past 30 years, the number of heart attacks has decreased due to changes in lifestyle and public awareness about the causes of heart disease. In addition, improved intensive-care facilities and new medications have decreased the chance of death after heart attacks from 30% to around 5% to 10%.

A *cardiologist* is a medical specialist trained to diagnose and treat heart diseases. A *cardiothoracic surgeon* is a specialist who performs heart (and lung) operations such as bypass surgery and valve replacements. There have been great medical advances in the area of heart disease, with new drugs and techniques available. Below will be a discussion of the most common heart diseases and a brief discussion of some treatments.

Heart Attacks

A heart attack occurs when blood flow to an area of the myocardium stops due to a narrowing in the coronary artery supplying that area of the heart. The symptoms of a heart attack are varied but include chest pain, shortness of breath, diaphoresis (sweating), nausea, vomiting, and arm pain or numbness. Unfortunately, nearly 30% of all heart attacks are "silent," meaning a person does not experience chest pain and does not know to seek medical attention. The chest pain of a heart attack is usually a substernal pressure or dull ache and has been described as feeling as if there were a band around the chest or an elephant sitting on the chest. Often this pain radiates into the left arm or to the jaw. Most sufferers deny that they are having a heart attack and blame heartburn or indigestion for their chest pain. When this happens, valuable minutes are lost in the treatment of the heart attack. On the other hand, not all chest pain comes from the heart, so other tools are needed to determine if the pain is cardiac in origin. Usually a heart attack is diagnosed with an ECG which shows which area of the heart is being injured (anterior or inferior wall, for example). In addition, blood tests that detect the release of cardiac enzymes from dead myocardial tissue are obtained every 8 to 12 hours to determine heart damage.

Atherosclerosis is a disease in which cholesterol plaques build up in the arteries, causing a narrowing in the vessel lumen. Once the narrowing reaches 70% of the vessel diameter, blood flow reaching the tissue is inadequate, and chest pain termed *angina* is experienced. Angina typically occurs with exertion when the oxygen demand of the heart exceeds the supply (which is inhibited by the cholesterol blockage). The pain usually resolves within minutes with rest, which changes the ratio of supply and demand. When a heart attack occurs, a blood clot forms in the area of narrowing because the blood flow in that area is sluggish and other metabolic factors encourage clotting. This blood clot now completely occludes the vessel. No blood reaches that area of the myocardium, and the tissue will die if flow is not restored with a few hours (Figure 10.1). That is why prompt medical care is essential in a heart attack. Within seconds, oxygen can be delivered and *nitroglycerine* tablets placed under the tongue to help get more oxygen to the myocardium. Nitroglycerine is a vasodilator, enlarging vessels so that more blood can get through. Drugs (like morphine) can be given to decrease the pain and alleviate anxiety; pain and anxiety cause

FIGURE 10.1

Myocardial infarction (heart attack). An area of stenosis (narrowing caused by atherosclerosis) may cause symptoms of angina. When a clot develops in a coronary artery, no blood flow reaches the myocardium supplied by that artery. If blood flow is not restored, the muscle dies resulting in a myocardial infarction.

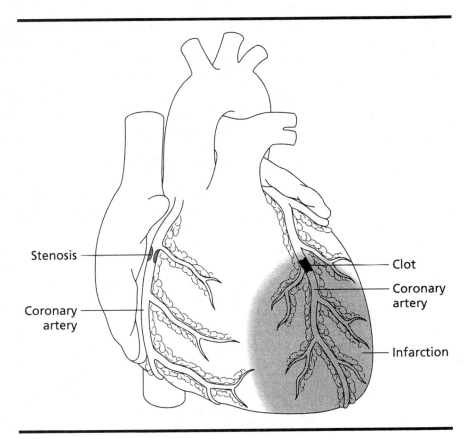

the blood pressure and heart rate to increase, putting even more stress on the heart.

Thrombolytic therapy is an effective treatment for heart attacks that has been developed in the past decade. Since the final step that occurs in the coronary artery during a heart attack is the formation of a blood clot, a medication that promptly dissolves the clot leads to restoration of blood flow to the myocardium. Three such "clot busters" are available in hospitals now, and all have been shown to significantly improve survival by opening up a blocked artery. Sometimes the heart attack can be aborted by giving these agents soon after chest pain starts. Studies have shown that the quicker thrombolytics are given, the better the outcome. Now the feasibility of delivering thrombolytic therapy "in the field" is being explored. Carrying these drugs in the ambulance and giving them even before the patient is transported to the hospital could make a huge difference in the number of lives saved. Nearly half of those who die from heart attacks do so before they can reach the hospital.

Death from a heart attack usually results from an abnormal heart rhythm or from pump failure, in which such a large area of the heart has been damaged that it cannot sustain muscle contraction. When abnormally slow heart rhythms are detected, medication or temporary electrical pacing keeps the heart rate up. When excessively fast, life-threatening rhythms develop (called ventricular tachycardia, or fibrillation), cardiopulmonary resuscitation and electrical defibrillation (electrical shocks delivered to the heart through paddles placed on the chest wall) are needed. You can do your part in helping save a life by taking a Red Cross or American Heart Association course in cardiopulmonary resuscitation. In CPR, artificial respirations and chest compressions can support the circulation until medical assistance arrives.

Risk Factors for Heart Disease

A risk factor is a condition that increases the likelihood of developing a disease. For example, smoking is a risk factor for lung cancer, and being a woman after menopause is a risk factor for osteoporosis. Likewise, there are risk factors for developing coronary artery disease which, are being male, old age, obesity, cigarette smoking, high blood pressure, diabetes mellitus, elevated cholesterol, a sedentary lifestyle, and a family history of coronary disease. These risk factors can be broken down into two major categories, modifiable risk factors and unmodifiable risk factors.

Risk factors that cannot be modified are your age, your sex, and your family history. Certain types of diabetes mellitus cannot be modified, but the most common type is affected by diet, body weight, and exercise, all of which can be modified by changes in lifestyle. Even sex has become a modifiable risk factor in a sense, because women have the same risk of coronary disease as men after menopause. Estrogen replacement may actually decrease this risk of heart disease in postmenopausal women. Estrogen has not been shown to decrease heart disease in men, however. As you can see, many risk factors can be modified by developing a healthy lifestyle. These will be discussed in the chapter of this manual on prevention and health maintenance.

Cardiac Tests

Several types of tests are used to detect heart diseases and determine the severity of heart damage. The most common one is the electrocardiogram (ECG), which shows heart rhythm and electrical conduction, suggests chamber sizes, can show an acute heart attack or areas of previous heart injury, and can reveal if certain areas of the heart are not getting enough blood. In an *exercise stress test*, the work of walking on a treadmill is gradually increased, placing more demand on the heart. If areas of the heart are not getting enough oxygen, characteristic changes on the ECG will occur suggesting the presence of coronary atherosclerosis. This test is not 100% accurate, and both false-positive and false-negative results occur.

A *holter monitor* is used to determine the presence of abnormal heart rhythms. ECG electrodes are placed on the chest, and a partial ECG tracing is recorded onto a cassette tape for 24 to 48 hours. A tape recorder is about the size of a small transistor radio is worn by the patient throughout daily activities.

In *nuclear imaging studies* a radioactive tracer is injected into the body, and images of the tracer in the heart are collected and processed by a computer. In one type of study, the ejection fraction of the heart can be obtained by determining how much of the tracer in the blood is pumped out of the heart with each contraction. In a nuclear stress test the tracer is injected at peak exercise and will be taken up in the heart only by areas receiving enough blood flow. If there is a blockage, the tracer cannot reach that area of the myocardium, and on the computer images, this area appears as a defect. This study can also be done on persons who cannot exercise on a treadmill by giving them a drug that sets up a stress situation. Nuclear imaging studies are more accurate than ECG stress tests but are still not perfect.

Cardiac catheterization, or *angiography (angiogram)*, is the most accurate means of detecting blockages in the coronary arteries. This procedure is done under local anesthesia and involves inserting a small sheath into the femoral artery in the groin. Then, a catheter can be advanced through the artery to the ascending aorta and engaged in the left or right coronary artery. An opaque x-ray dye is then injected through the catheter into the coronary artery, and the injection recorded on film. When the film is developed, the outlines of the vessels are seen, and the number, location, and severity of blockages are determined. In addition, a catheter can be advanced across the aortic valve and into the left ventricle, so that the ejection fraction can be determined by injecting dye into the beating ventricle. If it is not possible to enter from the groin, the brachial artery can be used to insert the catheters. A right heart catheterization involves advancing a catheter through the femoral vein, through the right atrium and ventricle, and into the pulmonary artery. No pictures are usually made, but important blood pressures and cardiac output can be measured.

Another important study, the *echocardiogram*, is discussed below.

Balloon Angioplasty

Once coronary artery disease is diagnosed, there may be several options for treatment. Medications can be given to return the oxygen supply-demand ratio toward a more favorable balance. No medications can reverse the cholesterol buildup directly, but lowering the blood cholesterol level with diet or medications and stopping smoking can gradually lead to a regression of atherosclerosis.

Another treatment option is *balloon angioplasty*. This procedure is very similar to a cardiac catheterization, but once the catheter is engaged in the coronary artery, a small, deflated balloon is passed over the wire to the point of the blockage. The balloon is inflated, and as it expands, the plaque is "smashed" out of the way. Initial success is greater than 90%, but a blockage recurs within six months about 30% of the time. If this happens, angioplasty can be done again.

New techniques for cleaning out arteries have been developed. An *atherectomy device* is a balloon with a small blade that actually shaves out the plaque and collects the plaque remnants in a little casing that is removed from the artery. *Laser angioplasty* is a technique in which a laser beam is radiated around the balloon in an attempt to "melt" the plaque into the side of the vessel and prevent a recurrence. A *cold laser beam* can be directed through a blockage, even a complete blockage, without first needing to pass the wire and balloon across the lesion. It may make a tunnel through the blockage so that a balloon can be advanced. The *rotational blade*, which is not yet available will hull out the artery blockage with a drill-like action.

In many cases, angina is completely relieved by one of these techniques, and medications are no longer needed. In other instances, the need for open heart surgery is eliminated, and activities can return to normal.

Coronary Artery Bypass Surgery

Coronary artery bypass grafting (CABG) is open heart surgery in which the blockages in the coronary arteries are bypassed by placing a piece of leg vein into the aorta and inserting the other end into the artery *beyond* the blockage (Figure 10.2). If two vessels are bypassed, it is a double bypass, and five (or possibly more) vessels can be bypassed. The mammary artery in the chest can be used instead of a vein to perform a bypass. The distal end of

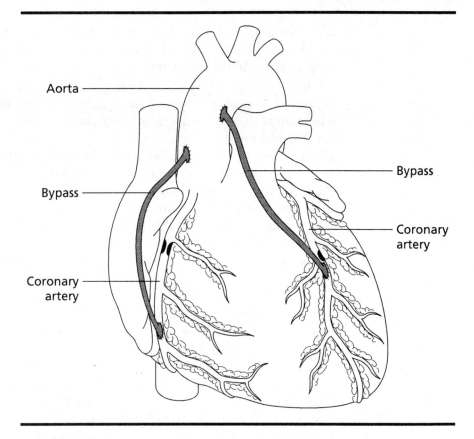

FIGURE 10.2
Coronary artery bypass grafting. Vein "grafts" taken from the leg are used to bypass the atherosclerotic blockage. The grafts are "sewn" into the aorta and then inserted into the coronary artery beyond the blockage.

the vessel is dissected free and inserted into the coronary artery. CABG is very effective in relieving chest pain, and in some instances survival is prolonged when surgery is performed. Unfortunately, the vein grafts are also susceptible to atherosclerosis and may become blocked. When this happens, another CABG can usually be done to restore adequate blood flow to the heart. Also, angioplasty or atherectomy can be performed on vein grafts as well.

Enlarged Hearts and Echocardiography

Two types of enlarged hearts exist: dilated hearts and hypertrophied hearts. Dilated, or balloon-type, hearts have thin walls and larger chambers. Hypertrophied hearts have thick walls and normal-sized or smaller chambers. Dilated hearts are caused most commonly by coronary artery disease and heart attacks; however, viral infections and undetermined factors may cause the heart to dilate as well. Dilated hearts may reach the point where systolic heart failure occurs because the myocardium is too thin and too weak to pump blood adequately.

Cardiac hypertrophy is usually caused by high blood pressure but can be caused by heart attacks, valve disease, or undetermined factors. In this condition the muscle of the heart thickens in an attempt to compensate for the need for greater blood delivery. This situation is analogous to the situation in skeletal muscles, which also hypertrophy when they are forced to exercise. In persons whose hypertrophy results from a disease process, the diastolic function (filling) of the heart is impaired, and a variety of problems results. It is interesting that endurance athletes develop cardiac hypertrophy, but this type of hypertrophy is not harmful, and their hearts are stronger and more efficient than before.

How is an enlarged heart detected? How are dilated hearts distinguished from hypertrophied hearts? The size of the heart is best determined by the use of sound waves. This technique is known as echocardiography (*echo* = sound; *cardio* = heart; *graphy* = writing). In echocardiography, a blunt probe that emits sound waves is placed on the chest wall and aimed at the heart. The sound waves "echo" off of the moving heart and create a picture of the heart on videotape that can be viewed by a physician. The chamber size and wall thickness can be determined from the videotape. This information allows the physician to differentiate between dilated and hypertrophied hearts. Echocardiography is used also to look at the flow of the blood through the heart and thus determine problems involving tight or leaky valves The sound waves can be "color-coded," which provides additional information. Echocardiography is not painful and provides a wealth of information about the size, dimensions, and functioning of the heart.

Heart failure is a disease in which adequate oxygen delivery to the tissues is not provided because the heart muscle is too weak (systolic failure) or because diastolic filling of the heart is impaired (diastolic failure). When heart failure develops, fatigue, shortness of breath, coughing, swelling of the lower extremities (edema), and the inability to sleep at night due to breathing problems occur. Diagnosis of heart failure is made on physical exam and usually confirmed with the aid of an echocardiogram. This common disorder affects two million people in the United States and contributes significantly to mortality, hospitalizations, and medical care. Unfortunately, medical treatment is only minimally effective in heart failure, and despite the best drug therapy, mortality remains high with this disease.

Artificial Hearts and Cardiac Transplantation

Heart transplantation is the most successful treatment for severe heart failure. When the heart muscle deteriorates to the point that a person cannot breathe comfortably at rest, even on the best available medications, a transplant is considered. Cardiac transplantation offers new hope to individuals who would otherwise die from heart failure. Thousands of persons die while waiting for a donor heart. In experienced centers, the survival rate after a transplant is greater than 90%, and without transplant, the survival rate is less than 20%.

An artificial heart is a mechanical pump that helps the heart deliver blood to the body. The artificial heart is a temporary bridge to support life until a transplant can be performed and is not designed to be a permanent heart replacement. A series of tubes divert blood from the heart to the mechanical pump and back to the circulation. The artificial heart is about the size of a two-drawer file cabinet and can be portable. Even so, a person with an artificial heart must remain in the hospital for close monitoring.

Two recent developments in the area of heart failure treatment are a muscle wrap and baboon heart transplantation. With the muscle wrap, the latissimus dorsi muscle is wrapped around the heart and stimulated to contract in synchrony with the heart, thereby augmenting the muscle force of contraction. Baboon heart transplantation for humans is experimental but could potentially save thousands of those who die while waiting for human donor hearts. Because of the huge emotional, financial, and social implications of heart transplantation, better preventive and therapeutic modalities deserve extensive research support.

Heart Defects

Heart defects are structural abnormalities, usually present at birth, that allow mixing of blood between the heart chambers. The most common are septal defects, in which there is a hole in the atrial septum or ventricular septum. *Atrial septal defects* may not be detected until adulthood, when symptoms of fatigue, shortness of breath, or abnormal heart rhythms occur. Sometimes they are incidental findings on an echocardiogram obtained for another reason. When identified, atrial septal defects should be repaired to prevent development of permanent problems. *Ventricular septal defects* are usually diagnosed in the newborn due to the presence of a loud murmur. Many defects will close on their own by age 4, but if they persist, repair should be done. Many other congenital defects allow abnormal mixing of blood. In certain cases, unoxygenated blood from the right heart is shunted to the left heart and delivered to the body. When this occurs, the baby has a blue discoloration due to the amount of deoxygenated blood circulating through the skin.

Artificial Valves

Thousands of people undergo *valve replacement* each year. Open heart surgery is performed and the abnormal valve is removed and replaced with an artificial valve. There are two kinds of artificial valves. One is made with metal and plastic parts, and the other is a valve taken from an animal heart (usually pig) and processed for insertion into a human heart. The metal valves usually last longer but have more problems with blood clots forming, so a blood thinner must be taken for life. Both types can get infected and lead to serious illnesses.

Who needs a valve replacement? Two types of valve problems can lead to malfunction of the heart. First, the valve may be too tight so that the flow of blood through the heart is obstructed. Second, a valve may be leaky and blood may actually flow the wrong direction between heart chambers. In either case, the delivery of blood to body tissues is compromised and may result in symptoms of fatigue, shortness of breath, irregular heart rhythms, and even collapse. A valve problem is diagnosed by listening to the heart with a stethoscope and detecting a *murmur*, an abnormal heart sound caused by the blood passing the valves. Not all murmurs indicate the presence of valve problems (some murmurs are innocent), but certain valve diseases will give a specific type of murmur (a leaky valve does not sound the same as a tight one). Once a murmur is heard, an echocardiogram can be used to determine the severity of the valve disease. There are no effective medications for correcting valve disease, but drugs can be given to relieve some symptoms and improve the ability of the heart to deliver blood. Ultimately, an abnormal valve causing significant problems will need to be replaced.

Irregular Heartbeat

Atrial fibrillation is a common problem in which the atria of the heart do not beat regularly. The rhythmic depolarization of the sinus node does not occur, and instead there is disorganized, spastic depolarization of the atria several times a second. When these rapid, sporadic impulses reach the atrioventricular node, they get conducted to the ventricles, causing a rapid and irregular heartbeat. (When the ventricles fibrillate, death occurs suddenly if the patient is not treated.) Persons with atrial fibrillation may be aware of a fluttering in the chest or may notice the irregular heartbeat by checking a pulse. Some people are not aware of the abnormal heartbeat, but have difficulty breathing or exercising. Atrial fibrillation is diagnosed on physical exam by taking the pulse, listening to the heart, and with an electrocardiogram. The ECG will show the lack of atrial P waves and the irregular rhythm of ventricular complexes.

Several factors can cause atrial fibrillation. Coronary artery disease or previous heart attacks, high blood pressure, and heart valve problems are primary cardiovascular diseases causing atrial fibrillation. Thyroid diseases in which too much thyroid hormone is produced will also cause it, as well as caffeine, nicotine, excess alcohol, and physical or emotional stress.

There are two major complications of atrial fibrillation. First, the heart rate may be so rapid (up to 200 beats per minute) that ventricular filling is compromised and leads to heart failure. Second, because the fibrillating atria are not pumping the blood, a blood clot may form in the atria. If it breaks loose, it could cause a stroke. Atrial fibrillation can often be treated with medication, but an electrical shock is sometimes delivered to the heart to restore sinus rhythm.

Pacemakers

A *pacemaker* is an electrical device that consists of a battery-operated generator and one or two wires. The generator is about half the size of a wallet and is inserted under the skin below one of the clavicles. The wires are connected to the generator and then placed (by way of the subclavian vein) into the right ventricle and, sometimes, into the right atrium (Figure 10.3). Then the electrical impulse produced by the generator can be transmitted through the wires to electrically stimulate the heart. The pacemaker can sense the heart's own electrical activity and will fire an impulse only when

FIGURE 10.3
Pacemaker. The pacemaker generator is placed under the skin. Wires (or leads) deliver the electrical impulse created by the generator to the right atrium and ventricle.

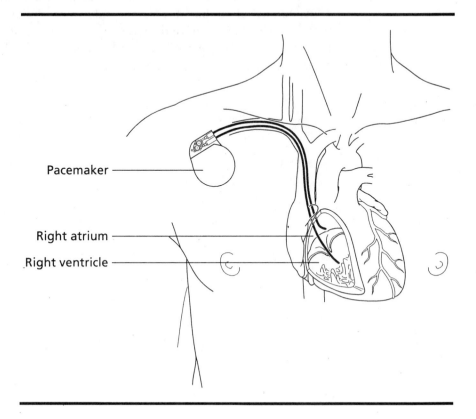

Pacemaker

Right atrium

Right ventricle

the heart fails to do so. Newer models can even be programmed so that the rate at which the pacemaker fires is determined by the amount of physical activity the person is doing as indicated by muscle activity or breathing patterns. A lithium battery drives the generator. It lasts 7 to 12 years depending of how frequently the pacemaker fires an impulse. Once the battery wears out, the generator is replaced and is connected to the existing wires.

Who needs a pacemaker? With age and some heart diseases, the natural pacemaker (sinus node) or conduction tissues (atrioventricular node and Purkinje fibers) in the heart dysfunction. When this happens, the heart rate may slow down severely or even stop altogether for a few seconds. This can cause a person to black out and may even lead to permanent damage or death. In these cases, a pacemaker is placed as a backup to sustain the rhythm of the heart.

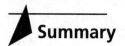

Summary

Valves, arteries, muscle, and electrical system of the heart are all susceptible to disease. There is a wide variety of diagnostic studies and treatment options available to persons with heart disease and many more in development. Coronary artery disease is the most common heart disease and is responsible for the greatest mortality among US men and women. Public education about cardiac risk factors and ways to modify these risk factors with lifestyle changes have decreased the incidence of this disease. Every person should take responsibility for his or her own health and make every effort to reduce the risk of heart disease.

11 Blood Vessels

CASE PRESENTATIONS

Mrs. Martin, 70, just returned from a long car trip to visit her children. She rode with her husband 12 hours in one day, stopping only for meals and gas. The following morning she felt pain and her right calf, which gradually got worse when she walked, and later that day she went to see her family doctor. Mrs. Martin had osteoarthritis of her knees, and her only medicines were an arthritis medication and estrogen replacement therapy. She told the doctor she had ridden in the car all day and, when asked, confessed to having worn her girdle that day.

On physical examination, the right calf appeared red, was tender to the touch, felt very hot, and was swollen, measuring 2 inches more in circumference than the left. She had normal movement in the right leg and had very minor arthritis pain in her knee. Her doctor told her that she had a blood clot in her leg and admitted her to the hospital to start treatment with a blood thinner. Mrs. Martin did not want to go to the hospital, but she agreed once her doctor had explained that without treatment, the clot could advance and break loose. If this happened, the clot could go to the lungs and cause serious breathing problems, even death.

Mr. Martin, 72, had pain in his right calf. His pain occurred several times a day when he was walking or climbing stairs. He usually walked slowly to try to prevent the pain from coming on, and any pain resolved within a few minutes if he stopped walking. Three months after returning from their trip, Mr. Martin developed a severe episode of pain in his right calf one evening while watching TV. The pain progressed until he could not tolerate it, and his wife drove him to the emergency room. Other than the excruciating leg pain, he felt fine, and he could not remember injuring his leg.

Mr. Martin had a history of high blood pressure but did not always take his medication. He also had an elevated cholesterol level and smoked cigarettes. His father and one brother died from a stroke.

On exam, his right leg appeared very pale, even bluish in color, and was cold to the touch. It was very painful but not swollen. He was having difficulty moving his foot and his toes. The doctor in the emergency room told Mr. Martin that he had a clot in his artery and that he could loose his leg if an emergency angiogram was not done. He was started on a blood thinner, and during the night the radiologist and vascular surgeon did the angiogram and gave a dose of a thrombolytic down the artery to dissolve the clot. The next morning, the pain was much better, and by the end of the week, he had bypass surgery done on his leg.

Questions

1. How were the Martins' lower-extremity blood clots different?
2. What factors contributed to Mrs. Martin's clot?
3. How was Mr. Martin's clot similar to a heart attack?
4. What is peripheral vascular disease, and what are the risk factors?

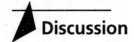 Discussion

Blood clots are common disorders. They can occur in the veins (*venous thrombosis*) or in the arteries. When an arterial occlusion occurs, it can be caused by thrombus (clot) in which underlying atherosclerosis causes a narrowing in the vessel and a *thrombus* forms in the narrowing (similar to what occurs with a heart attack). Arterial occlusions can also be caused by an *embolus*, a clot that is formed elsewhere in the body, breaks loose, and travels through the vasculature until it lodges in a vessel and obstructs blood flow. The body has a natural mechanism to dissolve blood clots, but when they occur in the great veins or in the arteries, clot dissolving medications are usually needed to prevent clot progression or to dissolve the clot quickly to return blood flow to the area.

The other vascular disease that is very common and causes significant medical problems is *hypertension* (high blood pressure), which will be discussed later.

Venous Thrombosis

Venous thromboses are common in the lower extremities. When a blood clot forms in the veins, the return of blood to the heart is blocked, and too much blood accumulates in the area usually drained by the vein. The result is swelling, pain, warmth, and redness in the area. These symptoms usually come on gradually as more and more blood accumulates, and elevation of the affected leg will provide relief by recruiting gravity and other venous routes to assist with the drainage.

Venous thromboses are caused by conditions in which venous blood flow is sluggish. This occurs with lack of activity, constrictive clothing, immobilization, and certain underlying medical conditions. Also, there are factors that contribute to blood clotting, such as the estrogen in birth control pills. Venous thromboses can be prevented by ensuring proper activity (especially when traveling long distances), wearing loose-fitting clothing, and giving small doses of blood thinners to persons who are bedridden or hospitalized. Users of birth control pills who smoke are much more likely to develop a clot than those who don't.

Once a thrombus forms, treatment involves giving blood thinners to prevent more clots from forming and giving the body a chance to dissolve the clot that is there. After initial treatment in the hospital, most persons must take a potent blood thinner called *warfarin* (once used as a rat poison) to prevent clots from forming again.

The most serious complication from a venous thrombosis occurs when it dislodges, travels through the veins to the right atrium and ventricle, and then becomes lodged in a pulmonary artery. This is called a *pulmonary embolus* and can be fatal. It appears that only clots in the deep veins in the leg embolize to the lungs. Thus, clots in the upper extremity and those of the superficial veins (including varicose veins) are treated conservatively with rest, elevation, and heat.

Peripheral Vascular Disease

The disease of *atherosclerosis*, which was discussed in the last chapter, is not limited to the coronary arteries but rather is a diffuse process that can involve "peripheral" arteries anywhere in the body (Figure 11.1). When atherosclerotic lesions are present in the carotid arteries, a stroke may occur. When these cholesterol plaques build up in the arteries of the legs, *claudication* is the predominant symptom. Claudication is very much like cardiac angina. With exercise, the oxygen demand in the legs increases, but the amount of oxygen delivery to the tissue is obstructed by the cholesterol plaques. The result is pain, often described as a cramp, which is relieved with rest, allowing the oxygen balance to compensate.

As with coronary disease, areas of narrowing in the peripheral vasculature are also prone to thrombus formation. When this occurs, the blood supply to the leg (for example) is completely occluded, and the tissues will start to die if it is not returned. Symptoms of severe pain and partial or complete loss of function have an acute onset. On examination, the extremity is cold and appears pale or even bluish in color. An *angiogram* is a study to diagnose and define the location and extent of the clot. As with a cardiac catheterization, a catheter is placed in the artery, and x-ray dye is injected to visualize the vessel. An angiogram can also be a therapeutic procedure; thrombolytic therapy can be delivered through the catheter to the site of the thrombus, thus dissolving the clot.

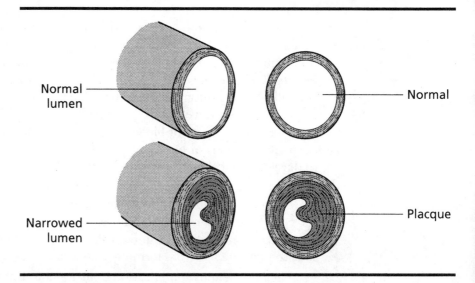

FIGURE 11.1
Atherosclerotic plaque in a blood vessel results in a narrowed lumen, which impedes blood flow and is susceptible to blood clot formation.

Treatment for peripheral vascular disease before clot formation is two-fold. First, better muscle conditioning will improve exercise tolerance, and second, a medication that makes the red blood cells more slippery so they move through the capillaries more easily results in better oxygen delivery. Nicotine makes the blockages worse, so stopping smoking is very important. Bypass surgery can also be performed on the peripheral vasculature. A vein or a synthetic graft (Dacron) can be sewn into the vessels so that the area of atherosclerotic blockage can be bypassed and blood flow restored to the extremity. However, these bypasses are not perfect and can also develop blockages and clots.

Fortunately, the body has its own mechanism for treatment of atherosclerosis. When one artery is not providing enough blood flow to the tissues, collateral arteries develop. They can increase the reserve flow significantly, and a person with even a total blockage may not have symptoms because the collateral vessels have been recruited and are delivering enough blood to the tissues.

Aneurysms And Malformations

Arterial *aneurysms* are dilatations, or enlargements, in an artery, usually caused by atherosclerosis and hypertension. These can be life threatening if they reach a certain size in the aorta because they could rupture. When aneurysms reach a certain size, the risk of rupture is so great that the vessel is repaired surgically, usually with a synthetic (Dacron) graft.

An *arteriovenous malformation* is a faulty connection in which the blood does not traverse the capillaries but flows directly from the artery to the vein. When this occurs, the veins dilate and may cause a cherry-colored mark on the skin that is present at birth. Depending on the location and severity of the malformation, surgical repair is sometimes indicated.

Raynaud's Disease

Vascular tone refers to the state of contraction or relaxation of the blood vessels. For example, when it is very cold outside, the vessels contract to prevent heat loss. Likewise, the vessels dilate with exercise to ensure adequate blood flow to exercising muscles. Each person has a given set point for vascular tone. This may in part explain why some people tolerate cold temperatures better than others.

Raynaud's disease is a condition in which the arteries of the digits undergo episodes of spasm (severe constriction) and probably reflects an abnormality with vascular tone. The spasm is precipitated by cold temperatures and emotional stress. Even entering an air-conditioned room in summer or taking food out of a freezer may precipitate an attack. When spasm occurs, it usually involves the fingers or entire hand(s) and is often bilateral. Symptoms resolve after about 15 to 20 minutes when the hands are warmed, often by running warm water over them. The symptoms of Raynaud's disease are severe pain, numbness, and tingling in the affected digit(s). Although symptoms are usually in the hands, the feet, ears, and nose are also affected.

A triphasic color pattern (white–blue–red) is characteristic of Raynaud's phenomenon. First, the hands become white when the vessel spasms and no arterial blood flows to the area. The blue phase occurs shortly thereafter as the deoxygenated venous blood leaks back into the empty capillaries. When the hands are warmed, there is an intense red phase as the artery opens and blood is pushed back into the capillaries.

Raynaud's disease can occur as a separate entity or be associated with other diseases. It is common in women aged 20 to 40. There is no specific treatment, but attacks can be prevented by keeping warm, eliminating emotional stress, not smoking, and avoiding certain drugs that precipitate arterial spasm.

Varicose Veins

Varicose veins are veins in the lower extremity that become dilated and prominently visible. There are two types of varicose veins, subcutaneous ("sunburst") varicose veins, which appear as small, blue spiders, and saphenous vein varicosities, which are long and tortuous. Usually, varicose veins are asymptomatic, however, aching and heaviness in the area may occur, as well as foot swelling at the end of a working day. Rarely, the vein will become inflamed, a condition called *thrombophlebitis*. This can be painful but usually resolves completely with rest, heat, elevation, and anti-inflammatory medication.

The cause of varicose veins is increased pressure in the venous system of the lower extremity. Varicose veins are more common in women, especially following the child-bearing years, as pregnancy impedes venous blood flow from the lower extremities. Tumors in the abdomen or conditions which cause excess straining will also lead to varicose veins.

Treatment for varicose veins is largely cosmetic. If discomfort occurs, support stockings may provide complete relief. When cosmetic treatment is desired, two techniques can be employed. First, the veins can be *sclerosed* (hardened) if they are small enough. This is usually done with the subcutaneous veins. An irritating substance is injected into the empty vein which is then compressed with an elastic wrap. Essentially the vein is scarred away. For larger veins, surgical removal (stripping) is required, often under general anesthesia. The recurrence rate after surgical treatment is about 10%, and usually additional sclerosing is needed to treat smaller veins.

Hypertension

Hypertension, or high blood pressure, is a major health problem in the United States and other developed countries. The magnitude of this problem is often underestimated because it is a "silent disease," meaning that persons with hypertension are without symptoms (asymptomatic) except in rare instances. Therefore, hypertension is diagnosed only in those persons who visit a medical facility and have their blood pressure taken. The U.S. incidence of hypertension is estimated at 10% to 20% of the general population but may be as high as 50% to 60% in certain populations (for example, urban, black, elderly females). This common problem can lead to significant cardiovascular disease and to death from heart attacks and strokes. Hypertension can sometimes be treated without medications, and with treatment the risks of complications caused by this disease are significantly reduced.

The definition of hypertension has been chosen to indicate a value at which the risk of cardiovascular disease is increased. Clinically, a diastolic pressure of more than 90 mm Hg and a systolic pressure of more than 140 mm Hg define hypertension. Because blood pressure is a variable that changes with activity, stress, and sympathetic tone (tension in the smooth muscle of vessel walls), one elevated blood pressure measurement alone should not be used to diagnose hypertension, especially in a doctor's office where stress is often an important factor. However, if one's blood pressure is found to be elevated, repeat measurements are mandatory. If blood pressure is elevated on three occasions, the hypertension should receive medical attention. Hypertension is classified as mild, moderate, or severe depending on the degree of elevation, and as the severity increases, the management must be more aggressive to prevent potentially catastrophic events.

The causes of hypertension in most cases are unclear. Hypertension of unknown origin is referred to as essential (primary) hypertension. This class of hypertension accounts for 90% to 95% of all cases. Since the causes are unknown, prevention and cure present real problems. However, treatment for this disease is very effective. Hypertension with an identifiable cause is called secondary hypertension. Secondary hypertension accounts for fewer than 10% of all cases. If the cause of hypertension can be diagnosed, it can often be cured by treating the underlying problem. Let us look more closely at secondary hypertension before returning to the more complex essential hypertension.

The cause of secondary hypertension in a patient is usually determined by using a careful history and physical examination along with added information obtained from simple laboratory studies. Kidney and endocrine abnormalities account for most cases of secondary hypertension. For example, disease in the renal arteries or in the kidney itself can cause hypertension. Endocrine diseases are rare, but oral contraceptive use is the most common hormonal cause of secondary hypertension. Hypertension develops in 5% of all women using oral contraceptives. If use is discontinued, about half of these women will have a return to normal blood pressure within six months. Age, kidney disease, obesity, and a family history of hypertension are risk factors that predispose women taking birth control pills to the development of hypertension. Some authorities believe that chronic alcohol abuse causes hypertension and that if alcohol use is discontinued, blood pressure will return to normal in about a week.

Essential hypertension is less understood than secondary hypertension. Risk factors contributing to its development include hereditary factors, obesity, smoking, salt intake, sedentary lifestyle, and stress. Identifying these risk factors is important, as modifications of them are sometimes effective in treatment. A variety of factors is involved in the regulation of blood pressure, and changes in any of these may contribute to hypertension. Sympathetic tone in blood vessels, blood vessel properties, kidney function, and hormones all affect blood pressure and may play varying roles.

The role of salt intake in hypertension is variable. The blood pressure of some hypertensive persons changes in correlation with salt intake. Sodium has been thought to be the key factor in salt-sensitive hypertension, but recent studies suggest a more important role of chloride and calcium in these persons. The mechanism by which salt affects blood pressure is unknown, but it may involve a defect of the plasma membrane in the regulation of sodium movements, or the kidney's ability to excrete sodium. Independent of the exact mechanism, it is clear that in some persons, salt restriction causes a marked lowering of blood pressure. However, salt intake may have no effect on blood pressure in other persons, and to say that all salt is bad is inappropriate.

The complications caused by long-standing hypertension fall into four main areas. 1) Cardiovascular disease. Hypertension has been recognized as a risk factor for the development of atherosclerosis, leading to heart attacks, peripheral vascular disease, and strokes. Heart failure can develop over time as the heart tires from pumping against this high pressure. 2) Central nervous system (CNS) disease. In persons with hypertension, the risk of having a CNS bleeding complication is increased. Hypertension makes the cerebral vessels more apt to rupture, resulting in bleeding into the area of the brain they supply. The result is a stroke that is clinically the same as one caused by a clot or blockage of the vessel. 3) Kidney dysfunction. Hypertension can cause damage to the kidneys, and even persons with a mild elevation in pressure will show some degree of renal damage. When hypertension coexists with diabetes, the risk of requiring kidney dialysis is increased. 4) Eye complications. Changes in vision may occur when vessels in the eye hemorrhage due to hypertension. A detached retina may also result, causing loss of sight. Of these four complications of hypertension, the most life-threatening is cardiovascular diseases. Persons with other risk factors for cardiovascular diseases should monitor and control their blood pressures closely.

The treatment of hypertension is multifaceted, and a broad approach to lowering blood pressure can be very effective and well tolerated. Measures that do not involve medication should be attempted before medical therapy is instituted, because they can be quite effective, and medications have side effects. (It is challenging to convince people to take a medication that may make them feel worse for a disease that is asymptomatic.) These measures include weight reduction, salt restriction, increased physical activity, stopping smoking, alcohol reduction, and biofeedback techniques. If these measures fail to achieve a desirable blood pressure, medications are required. The use of antihypertensive drugs is almost an art, as there are many classes of agents available and different agents within each class. These medications can be used alone or in combination, as needed. Several classes of antihypertensive medications will be briefly discussed to aid your understanding of hypertension and its treatment.

Diuretics lower blood pressure by decreasing blood volume through urinary excretion of fluid. Because many diuretics also cause renal losses of ions, sodium and especially potassium need to be monitored in persons taking diuretics. **Beta-adrenergic blockers** work by decreasing cardiac output, renin activity, and sympathetic tone. Side effects include gastrointestinal complaints, fatigue, sedation, and sexual impotence and may necessitate discontinuation of therapy. Other agents alter sympathetic tone by acting on either the central or peripheral nervous system, but these are more complicated and are used less commonly. **Vasodilators** act directly on blood vessels to relax smooth muscle and decrease resistance. Headaches, an increased heart rate (tachycardia), and heart palpitations are the most common side effects of vasodilators. **Calcium channel blockers** have been highly effective in lowering blood pressure by blocking the entry of calcium into cells. This decreases smooth muscle contractility, sympathetic tone, and cardiac output. **Angiotensin converting enzyme (ACE) inhibitors** block the final step in the renin-angiotensin system and cause vasodilation. In summary, a number of antihypertensive drugs exist, and when one class of agents is not effective in controlling blood pressure, another class can be tried alone or in combination with the previous agent. Medical therapy does not eliminate the need to modify factors that may contribute to hypertension, as these changes will also decrease the risk of developing complications.

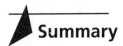 **Summary**

Vascular diseases may be caused by atherosclerosis, blood clots , vessel spasm, or congenital malformations. Hypertension is the most common "vascular disease". Hypertension is an asymptomatic disease yet it contributes to significant complications including heart disease, strokes, kidney disease, and eye problems. Medication may be needed to control hypertension, but many persons can reduce body weight, quit smoking, exercise regularly, and make dietary changes to adequately control blood pressure.

12 Blood

CASE PRESENTATIONS

Sharon and Michelle, both 34, went to the same aerobics class. For several months both had been feeling fatigued and had less energy to exercise. Gradually, they noticed being short of breath with light activity, and their friends commented that they looked pale. Eventually, both went to their gynecologists for a routine pelvic exam and mentioned their symptoms. Both had normal physical exams, and blood tests were drawn.

Sharon's doctor called her back and told her she had anemia (a low level of red blood cells) and recommended that she liberalize her diet to include iron-rich foods and begin taking iron supplements.

Michelle's gynecologist asked her to come in for another appointment, and when she did, she found out that she had leukemia and was referred to another physician for further tests and treatment.

Questions

1. Why did these two women have the same symptoms but such different diseases?
2. What causes anemia?
3. Can anemia be prevented?
4. What is leukemia, and what is the prognosis of this disease?

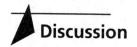

Discussion

Hematology is the study of the blood, blood-forming tissues, and the diseases that affect them. A *hematologist* is a physician who specializes in blood diseases and their treatment. Generally, hematological diseases can be divided into three main categories: anemias, disorders of white blood cells, and clotting disorders. Examples of each of these will be discussed below.

Symptoms or physical exams usually offer little insight into in blood disorders, but a simple blood test provides a wealth of information. When a *CBC* (complete blood count) test is taken, several pieces of information are obtained. First, the concentration, number, size, and appearance of the red blood cells (erythrocytes) are measured. *Anemia* is diagnosed by finding a low concentration of red cells, and the cause can also be suggested. For example, if one does not get enough iron in the diet or has bleeding, the red cells are not only decreased but also appear very small (Figure 12.1). If the anemia stems from a lack of vitamin B_{12}, the number is decreased but the cells are excessively large and have many different shapes. The platelet count is important to ensure proper clotting. Platelets can be decreased by certain cancers or by chemotherapy, and there can be primary abnormalities of the platelets.

The leukocyte count and differential are very important, for two major reasons. First, leukemia is detected by observing a high leukocyte level and detecting premature cells in the peripheral blood (see Figure 12.1). This blood test can also be used to determine the response of leukemias to treatment. Second, infections elicit a particular type of leukocyte response, which can be detected with a CBC. With bacterial infections, the neutrophil count is markedly elevated, but with viral infections, it may be normal, and the lymphocyte count will be up. In fact, mononucleosis (a viral disease that plagues college students) was named such because of the elevated monocyte count (now referred to as atypical lymphs) that accompanies the infection.

The bone marrow is another place where information can be obtained about hematological diseases. Since the majority of the blood elements are derived from cells in the bone marrow, sampling and examining this tissue yields much information, especially about cancers. A *bone marrow biopsy* is a procedure in which a large-bore needle is inserted into the bone marrow in the iliac crest. When the needle is withdrawn, a sample of tissue is taken and prepared for microscopic examination. This study can also be used to follow response to leukemia therapy.

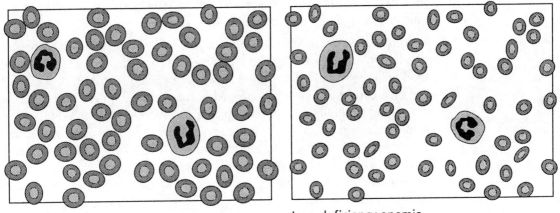

Normal blood smear

Iron-deficiency anemia

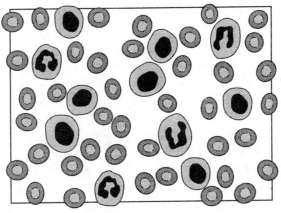

Chronic lymphocytic leukemia

FIGURE 12.1
Histological blood smears. In iron-deficiency anemia, compared with normal blood, the erythrocytes are smaller and fewer in number. The smear demonstrating leukemia shows increased lymphocytes that are poorly differentiated crowding out erythrocytes.

Anemia

Anemia can be measured by determining the number of red cells in the blood, by measuring the amount of hemoglobin in the blood, or by the proportion of red cells in the blood (called the hematocrit). The symptoms associated with anemia are usually vague and include fatigue, weakness, shortness of breath with exertion, and paleness. The physical exam is generally unremarkable except for pale skin tone and mucous membranes. If the anemia is severe, the heart rate may be increased and the blood pressure decreased. Sometimes there is also a heart murmur that resolves when the anemia is corrected. Anemia is easily diagnosed with a blood test and the values obtained can be used to follow treatment as well. There are many causes of anemia, and a few will be discussed below.

Iron-deficiency anemia is common. It results when the body's stores of iron are depleted, resulting in inadequate iron to make hemoglobin for red blood cells. It is caused by blood loss, lack of adequate dietary intake of iron, or a combination of the two. Men have more iron reserves than do women and generally do not develop anemia as often. Also, blood loss must occur over a long period (or be quite severe) before anemia develops. Young women who are menstruating and are on diets that do not include iron-rich foods will often develop anemia. In this case, the treatment is to increase the amount of iron in the diet, and occasionally iron tablets are given. Another common cause of iron-deficiency anemia is stomach ulcers. Blood is gradually lost through the stools. In any middle-aged person with iron-deficiency anemia and blood in the stools, a search for cancer of the colon should be pursued, as this is another common cause of blood loss.

There are also hereditary diseases that cause anemia. In sickle-cell anemia, a disease primarily affecting blacks, the B chain of hemoglobin has an abnormal animo acid. Under normal conditions, the abnormal B chain can bind to iron, but whenever the amount of oxygen in the blood is reduced, the B chain becomes disfigured. The red cells also become deformed, clump together, and are destroyed in the blood. This process of "bursting" red blood cells is called *hemolysis* (*hemo* = blood; *lysis* = split). Another inherited anemia is called thallasemia. The underlying problem in thallasemia is a genetic defect in which not enough of a hemoglobin chain is produced by the cells. Some types of this disease are fatal in childhood.

Hemoglobin and iron are not the only components needed for erythrocyte production. Deficiencies of certain vitamins (B_{12} and folate) can cause abnormal production of red cells. Liver disease, excessive alcohol consumption, and disorders in the bone marrow will also lead to abnormal erythrocytes, which appear unusually large on the blood smear. Correcting the underlying cause of the anemia will result in normal red cell counts.

Blood Transfusions

When anemia is severe or when there has been a large amount of blood loss (as with major trauma from an automobile accident), red blood cells must be replaced more quickly than the bone marrow can produce them to deliver enough oxygen to the tissues. A blood transfusion is a safe and effective means of delivering red cells into the blood.

When blood is donated for medical use, each unit is processed to separate the erythrocytes, platelets, and plasma. When excessive bleeding occurs, a unit (or more) of "packed red cells" is transfused. This transfusion contains mostly erythrocytes so that a concentrated boost of red cells is given. Plasma can further be processed to remove clotting factors or can be given directly as a plasma infusion. Platelets are given when the platelet numbers in the blood are so low that spontaneous bleeding occurs.

A transfusion is given through an intravenous catheter directly into a vein. Before the transfusion is given, the donor blood is carefully matched with the recipient's blood to prevent an immune transfusion reaction in which antibodies attack the antigens on the blood cells. In experienced hospital laboratories and blood banks, the risk of receiving a mismatched unit of blood is very small. Likewise, with predonation screening and careful testing procedures, the risk of acquiring AIDS from a transfusion today is also very small, although the risk does increase in large cities, where this disease is more common. The final risk of a blood transfusion is that of contracting hepatitis. Viral hepatitis is caused by a virus carried in the blood and can be spread through blood products. Again, careful screening is always done, but unfortunately, there is a period during which the virus is in the blood but cannot be detected. The risk of hepatitis is greater than the risk of AIDS or a mismatch and can lead to serious liver problems.

Hemophilia

Hemophilia is a hereditary clotting disorder in which a factor in the clotting cascade is lacking. The result is the inability to form a clot, even when a minor injury occurs, and massive, even fatal, bleeding results. The most common type of hemophilia is the lack of Factor VIII. The gene for this clotting factor is carried on the X sex chromosome, so that males are nearly exclusively affected. Christmas disease is a less common type of hemophilia. The missing factor is Factor IX, and the consequences can be just as fatal. The treatment for hemophilia is replacement of the lacking clotting factor, which is extracted from donor blood plasma. Unfortunately, several pints of blood must be pooled to provide enough of the missing factor, and the risk of infection with AIDS and hepatitis is greatly increased.

Leukemia

Leukemia is the leading cause of death by cancer in children under 15 years old and the sixth leading cause of cancer deaths in adults. Leukemia is a malignancy of the leukocytes in which they divide at a rapid, uncontrolled rate in the bone marrow. The symptoms are insidious, and the proliferation in the marrow does not usually cause pain. Rather, the symptoms are related to the affects of the malignant cells crowding out the normal marrow components, with resultant anemia, bleeding from lack of platelets, and infections that the normal white cells cannot fight off. Also, the liver, spleen, and lymph nodes may become noticeably enlarged as they become engorged with these malignant cells that accumulate in these organs as the leukocytes circulate. Fever and weight loss are also common symptoms of leukemia.

When one of these symptoms occurs, a CBC blood test is obtained and nearly always shows the anemia or lack of platelets. It will also show the excessive number of leukocytes in the blood, many of which are in immature forms. Even though leukemia can be diagnosed by the blood smear, the underlying abnormality is in the bone marrow, and a bone marrow biopsy is performed to determine which cell type has gone awry.

Leukemias are classified based on which cell type is malignant (lymphocyte or myelocyte) and whether the onset is acute or chronic. Acute leukemias account for more than half of leukemias and typically have a rapid, fatal outcome if not treated (survival for only a few months). Chronic leukemias progress more slowly, and survival without treatment is often two to three years.

The treatment for leukemias depends on the type of leukemia and the age of the patient. Chemotherapy is given to achieve a *remission*, which occurs when all the malignant cells have been irradicated from the bone marrow. Once remission is achieved, a bone marrow transplant should be considered to achieve a cure of the disease. If this cannot be done, the leukemia cells are likely to appear again. Remission can usually be achieved more than once, but each time this is more difficult. Death usually results from bleeding (due to lack of platelets), infection (lack of effective white cells), or metabolic disorders.

Bone Marrow Transplantation

Bone marrow transplantation is a novel approach that has revolutionized the treatment of many leukemias, some other cancers, and hematologic diseases. The advances in this area have proceeded rapidly, and bone marrow transplantation is now a well-accepted, conventional treatment for many of these disorders. For example, certain genetic disorders resulting in immunological deficiencies or inadequate production of red blood cells can be cured if the genetically deranged marrow is destroyed by irradiation, chemotherapy, or both. Following destruction of the defective native marrow, healthy marrow from a compatible donor is transplanted into the bones, where it regenerates and supplies the host with normal marrow elements. In addition to genetic disorders, some acquired disorders result in bone marrow failure. These may also be effectively treated with bone marrow transplantation. The long-term survival in these groups of patients is 50% to 75%; without bone marrow transplantation, their expected mortality would be near 100%.

The most experience with using bone marrow transplantation for the treatment of malignancies has been obtained with leukemia patients. Bone marrow transplantation has become accepted as the preferred means of treatment for people with chronic myeloid leukemia. The use of transplantation involves giving lethal doses of radiation and chemotherapy during remission to destroy all the malignant cells and any potential stem cells in the marrow that may reproduce the leukemic cell line. This treatment also destroys normal marrow cells and is incompatible with life, as one cannot live without marrow elements. Thus, the marrow must be replaced by transplantation. In cancers other than leukemia, the malignancy may not directly involve the bone marrow. However, doses of chemotherapy and radiation large enough to destroy all tumor cells destroy the bone marrow as well. (These agents have a much greater effect on rapidly dividing tissue such as marrow and tumors than on other types of tissue.) Bone marrow transplantation allows these doses to be given.

Bone marrow is obtained from a donor by multiple biopsies of the marrow in the iliac crest. The marrow is processed and administered to the patient via intravenous infusion. The circulating marrow cells settle out in the medullary cavities of bones, where they regenerate. Within two to four weeks, indications of the transplanted marrow appear, as evidenced by increases in the hematocrit, the number of platelets, and the white blood cell count. During the two- to four-week waiting period, the patient is supported as needed to prevent severe anemia (by red blood cell transfusions), bleeding (by platelet transfusions), and infections (by antibiotics, white blood cell transfusions, and sometimes antibody preparations). Sterile conditions are strictly observed to prevent introduction of microorganisms to the patient.

In certain malignancies, "autologous" bone marrow transplantation has had much success. In autologous transplantation, the marrow of the patient is harvested during remission when no malignant cells are thought to be present. This marrow is then frozen and sometimes treated in a way that destroys any cancer cell line. With this marrow "in the bank," treatments can be given to eliminate the cancer from the body. (These treatments also destroy the marrow.) When treatment is complete, the patient's own marrow is given back. This means of transplantation is preferred whenever possible, because it does not produce problems with rejection or graft-versus-host complications.

As techniques improve and treatment regimens become more sophisticated, bone marrow transplantation may play an even more important role in the treatment and cure of many diseases. Depending on the specific disease and the condition of the patient at the time of transplantation (most patients are quite ill with infections, anemia, or bleeding), 60% to 90% of patients survive the transplantation. A portion of the survivors will have delayed complications of infections, rejections, or graft-versus-host disease. However, nearly all of these patients would have died from their disease without bone marrow transplantation.

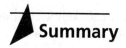

Summary

Erythrocytes, platelets, leukocytes, and clotting elements each perform important functions which can be altered by disease. Anemia can readily be diagnosed by a blood smear, but several other tests may be needed to determine the cause of anemia and initiate appropriate therapy. Platelet and clotting factor deficiencies can lead to serious bleeding disorders. Leukemias are caused by excessive, uncontrolled production of leukocytes. Blood transfusions are life-saving measures performed to replace cells or clotting factors in the circulation. Likewise, bone marrow transplantation has offered new hope for persons with malignant diseases.

13 Lymphatics and the Immune System

CASE PRESENTATIONS

Steve, 28, began noticing a sore throat and fever during work. That evening he felt achy all over and had a painful, swollen area on each side of his neck. He took some aspirin and went to see his company doctor in the morning because his symptoms had worsened. His doctor told him he had a strep throat and prescribed an antibiotic. When Steve asked about his neck, he was told he had inflamed, reactive lymph nodes. The bacterial infection in his throat was causing the lymph nodes to produce cells to fight the infection. Steve's lymph nodes remained very swollen and sore for a couple of days and then resolved totally.

Steve's older brother, 31, also noted a swelling in his neck. He did not have a sore throat or fever and generally felt well. The swelling was not painful but persisted several weeks, so he saw his company doctor. On physical exam, his throat was not infected, but he had swollen, nontender lymph nodes. The doctor recommended a biopsy, and the results confirmed a lymphoma. Steve's brother was referred to an oncologist for further tests and treatment.

Questions

1. How are reactive lymph nodes different from lymphoma?
2. What role does the lymphatic system play in fighting infection?
3. How do Steve and his brother differ in prognosis?
4. Why was Steve given antibiotics for his infection?

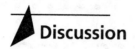

Discussion

The immune system is responsible for fighting off infections in the body. Most of the time, the immune system is able to irradicate the infection without assistance. This is true of most viral infections and a few bacterial infections. However, sometimes *antibiotics* are needed to help the immune system clear the invading organisms. Antibiotics are chemical compounds that either kill the organisms or prevent their growth, allowing the immune system to destroy the organisms. There are several antibiotics available for oral and intravenous use, and each antibiotic is effective only against specific organisms. In other words, the antibiotic used to treat strep throat is not effective against a urinary tract infection. An *infectious disease specialist* is a physician who has undergone training in the diagnosis and treatment of infectious diseases and other diseases of the immune system. An *oncologist* is a physician who specializes in cancer diagnosis, prevention, and treatment.

There are two major types of disease that directly involve the immune system. First, *autoimmune diseases* are ones in which the body inappropriately makes antibodies that attack its own tissues. Second, *acquired immunodeficiency syndrome (AIDS)* is caused by a virus that attacks certain immune cells so that the body cannot fight off infections and certain cancers. Both diseases can be devastating and fatal. *Lymphoma* is a malignant tumor composed of lymphocytes, usually in the lymph nodes and other lymphatic tissues. These diseases will be discussed below.

Lymph Nodes and Infection

The lymph nodes are the site of lymphocyte proliferation and differentiation. When a localized infection occurs, the bacteria are drained via the lymphatics to the lymph nodes, where the bacterial antigens are presented to the lymphocytes to induce antibody production and lymphocyte proliferation. The reaction may cause the lymph nodes to enlarge and become tender, a symptom we have all experienced. As the body destroys the infection, the lymph nodes return to normal and stand ready for the next infection.

The groups of lymph nodes that become active point to the area of infection. For example, ear infections typically recruit the lymph nodes behind the ear and in the posterior neck, where as sexually transmitted infections will cause lymph nodes in the groin to react. In certain skin and tissue infections of the extremities, the lymphatic themselves may become inflamed and a develop a red, streaking appearance up the arm or leg. The lymph nodes will also become involved and can be quite painful. Again, these symptoms all resolve with appropriate treatment, and no permanent damage results.

Lymphoma

Lymphomas are solid tumors composed of lymphocytes proliferating in lymphatic tissue, usually lymph nodes. A lymphoma possesses the malignant property of metastasis, and although it originates in an isolated lymph node area, the tumor may spread to other lymph nodes, the liver, the spleen, and even bone marrow and blood, resulting in a clinical picture similar to leukemia. Even before malignant lymphocytes invade bone marrow, infections are common due to a compromised immune system, and some of these infections can be fatal.

Lymphomas are classified into two main groups based on the histological presence or absence of the Reed-Sternberg cell (a large, multinucleated cell). When Reed-Sternberg cells are seen in biopsy specimens, Hodgkin's lymphoma is diagnosed. The significance of the Reed-Sternberg cell is not known, but clinically, Hodgkin's lymphoma behaves differently from non-Hodgkin's lymphoma (NHL) and responds differently to therapy.

Hodgkin's lymphoma is divided into four histological types, but they have little relevance to the clinical course or outcome of the disease. Rather, the extent of the spread of disease is the more important determinant of clinical behavior. In limited disease, treatment with radiation results in an 85% cure rate. Chemotherapy is required to threat widespread disease; in these cases, remission rates of 70% to 80% can be achieved, with long-term survival rates of up to 60%. Newer chemotherapy regimens boast even better remission rates, and the combination of chemotherapy and radiation therapy is particularly effective.

Unlike Hodgkin's lymphoma, NHLs are classified by histological types that do have clinical prognostic implications. In other words, in NHL, the extent of the disease is less critical than the tissue type that is involved. In favorable types, patients may live seven or eight years without any treatment, although about one-third of these lymphomas advance to more aggressive tumors, and the prognosis deteriorates. Even with radiation and chemotherapy, a cure is not usually achieved, but remissions can be induced. In aggressive types of NHL, despite chemotherapy and radiation therapy, the long-term survival rate is only 50% to 60%.

Allergies and Anaphylaxis

Allergies are a common plague of all ages. Although they are not life threatening, the symptoms are quite annoying and can compromise one's abilities. An allergic reaction is the immune system's response to a foreign antigen called an allergen. When one is exposed to the allergen, a hypersensitivity reaction occurs triggered by immunoglobulin E, lymphocytes and monocytes. One allergen—poison ivy—was discussed in relation to dermatitis and is an excellent example of an allergic reaction involving the skin. Insect bites fall into the same category. Most allergens are airborne plant pollens, dusts, and molds. These substances provoke the same allergic reaction in the nasal mucosa, airways, and eyes. This reaction leads to itching, copious secretions, and swelling of the membranes. Persons with allergies to certain plant products typically have seasons in which allergies are most severe. For example, ragweed pollens are prolific in late summer and early fall and last until the first freeze. Other plants, especially desert plants, produce annoying pollens in the mid- and late spring.

Treatments of allergies are diverse, depending on the allergen and type of reaction. For allergic rhinitis (hay fever, inflammation of the nasal mucosa), antihistamines and nasal sprays are most effective. If asthma results, inhalers, antihistamines, and cortisone-like drugs may be needed. Allergy shots can be given in which small amounts of the allergen are injected so that the immune mechanisms become desensitized to the allergen. This can be effective when a specific allergen(s) is identified.

The most severe allergic reaction is anaphylaxis. This is a systemic, widespread allergic reaction that can be fatal if not treated promptly. The symptoms of anaphylaxis are difficulty breathing due to airway obstruction and collapse due to vessel dilatation such that adequate blood pressure is not maintained. The most common allergens that cause anaphylaxis are antibiotic medications and insect venoms in wasp or bee stings. The treatment for anaphylactic shock is prompt opening of the airway by giving epinephrine and antihistamines. Sometimes an incision must be made at the base of the neck into the trachea (a tracheostomy) to get air into the lungs. Cortisone-like medications (usually prednisone) are also given to prevent inflammation, but these drugs take longer to act. Persons with known allergic reactions to bee and wasp stings often carry a "bee sting kit" containing epinephrine, antihistamine, and prednisone so that they can initiate treatment rapidly.

Autoimmune Diseases

Autoimmune diseases are caused by the body misinterpreting its own proteins and tissue components as foreign substances. When this occurs, immune complexes are either formed in the tissues or are formed in the blood and deposited in the tissues, usually in capillaries or arterioles. In other words, the body's defense mechanisms attack its own tissues. The spectrum of autoimmune diseases is broad and some are quite severe and disabling. Myasthenia gravis, as mentioned earlier, is an autoimmune disease in which antibodies bind the acetylcholine receptors in the neuromuscular junction. This causes muscle weakness, typically affecting smaller muscles. Also mentioned was rheumatoid arthritis in which autoantibodies cause arthritis and affect other connective tissues in the body. Rheumatoid arthritis can be a crippling disease. Three other diffuse autoimmune diseases will be mentioned below.

Systemic lupus erythematosus is a chronic inflammatory disease that affects many organs. Ninety percent of patients are female, and the disease is more common among blacks. This disease is very serious: only 10% of treated patients will have a long-lasting remission, and only 70% of patients survive for ten or more years after being diagnosed. Skin and joint involvement are common, but abnormalities in the blood, kidneys, and nervous system are the most severe problems. Other systems are also involved, although usually to lesser degrees. The treatment of systemic lupus erythematosus involves anti-inflammatory medications such as corticosteroids and a number of supportive measures such as physical therapy. To date there is no cure, and no medications are effective in significantly altering the progression of the disease. Different cytotoxic (cell-killing) drugs have been used in treatment, but they have many undesirable side effects. These agents are used in patients with life-threatening complications who have not responded to corticosteroids. The leading causes of death in systemic lupus erythematosus are renal failure and infections.

Scleroderma (*scler* = hard; *derm* = skin) is an uncommon disease characterized by tough, leathery skin. This disease results partially from increased collagen production. Inflammation and collagen deposition are most notable in the skin, kidneys, lungs, heart, and digestive tract. The result is a "stiffening" of these tissues, with the resulting loss of proper function. Scleroderma is a slowly progressive disease, affecting females more frequently than males. The severity and progression of the disease are quite variable, and although symptomatic treatment (treatment of symptoms rather than causes of the disease) has had some success, no medications have been proven effective in preventing the progression of the disease. The survival rate ten years after diagnosis is only 20%, and death is caused by heart, kidney, or lung complications.

Dermatomyositis is a rare syndrome caused by an inflammatory reaction in skin and skeletal muscle tissue. The clinical features include skin lesions, rashes, and muscle weakness. Females are affected more commonly than males, and there is an association with cancer in some types of the disease. Although muscle and skin involvement is the hallmark of this disease, the kidneys, heart, and lungs are also affected. Corticoteroids and cytotoxic drugs appear effective in treatment (50% of patients show complete recovery), but relapses are common. Seventy-five percent of patients survive for five or more years after diagnosis.

Acquired Immunodeficiency Syndrome

Acquired immunodeficiency syndrome (*AIDS*) is a devastating disease affecting millions of people worldwide. AIDS was first noted in 1981 when a rare type of pneumonia was reported among homosexual men, followed by a report of a rare cancer, Kaposi's sarcoma, also in gay men. Over the past decade, thousands in the United States and millions around the world have the disease we now know as AIDS, and millions more are infected with the deadly virus that causes the disease.

AIDS is caused by the *human immunodeficiency virus (HIV)*, but not all persons infected with HIV have AIDS. A better understanding of the course of the disease will help clarify that point. When a person first becomes infected with HIV, symptoms are usually mild and resemble those of a cold or the flu, usually lasting a couple of weeks. This initial infection (the virus is infecting the body's cells) is then followed by a period that is usually asymptomatic. This period in which a person has no symptoms but is infected (and therefore can spread the disease) typically lasts eight to ten years. This is then followed by a period in which nonspecific symptoms occur, including fatigue, fever, weight loss, rash, or minor infections, usually in the mouth. This nonspecific period is termed *AIDS-related complex (ARC)* and heralds the impending AIDS disease complex. The disease AIDS is defined by the presence of HIV infection and specific symptoms related to infectious diseases, cancers, severe weight loss, persistent fever, diarrhea, or neurological abnormalities. It appears likely that all persons with HIV infections will go on to develop AIDS unless new treatments are developed.

HIV cannot be detected in the blood, but antibodies against the virus can be. It may take up to six months to produce the antibodies, but the potential for spreading the virus is present. The initial testing is done with an *ELISA* test, but this can yield false positive results. Therefore, all positive tests are rechecked using a more sensitive test called a *western blot*. Pretest counseling is advised, and anonymous testing is available at many public health centers. Again, testing positive for HIV is not the same as having AIDS, but it is quite likely that AIDS will develop over the years.

HIV is found in the blood and in body secretions, mainly in semen and vaginal secretions. The three modes of transmission of the virus are through sexual activity, blood contamination, and from mother to fetus. Transmission through the blood is common among intravenous drug abusers who share contaminated needles. Even with small amounts of blood on the needle, the virus present is injected directly into the bloodstream and is highly infectious. Hemophiliacs also acquire HIV infections through the blood products given to replace clotting factors. Although the risk of infection through blood transfusions has been nearly eliminated through donor screening and blood testing, the risk of AIDS with a blood transfusion is 1 in 40,000 in large cities with a high AIDS population.

Sexual contacts are another way in which HIV is spread, and this mode of transmission is the primary means of infection in homosexual men. However, AIDS is not just a disease of homosexual men, and in fact the number of new HIV infections in this population is decreasing. Unfortunately, HIV infection in the United States is on the rise in heterosexuals due to sexual transmission. In Africa, heterosexual contact is the primary means of infection, and AIDS is a huge medical problem in several African and Asian countries.

Prenatal transmission of HIV from mother to fetus results in children with AIDS, and approximately one-third of infected mothers pass the virus on to their children in this way. HIV is *not* spread through household contact, touching, hugging, or kissing.

The primary problem with HIV infection that leads to AIDS is a lack of cell mediated immunity. HIV infects the helper T-lymphocytes and destroys them as the virus replicates in the cells. Without this line of defense, the body is susceptible to infections that usually do not cause disease. (The normal defense mechanisms usually destroy the infection.) These infections are called *opportunistic infections* because they take advantage of a compromised immune system. The most common opportunistic infection is *pneumocystis carinii*, an organism that causes pneumonia. Nearly 80% of AIDS patients will develop this type of pneumonia, which is difficult to treat and usually recurs. Viruses and tuberculosis also cause severe illnesses and can lead to death in AIDS patients. Unfortunately, many antibiotics are not effective in treating opportunistic infections, and unusually high doses of antibiotics must be given, which often cause severe side effects. Also, these infections can recur easily once antibiotics are stopped, so many persons must stay on these medications indefinitely. Opportunistic infections are often the cause of death in persons with AIDS, but new advances are being made in the treatment of these diseases.

Another result of HIV infection is increased occurrence of cancers, especially Kaposi's sarcoma, a tumor of endothelial cells. Kaposi's appears as deep blue or purple nodules on the skin and can metastasize in the body, typically to the GI tract or lungs. These tumors can bleed easily, and if this occurs in the GI tract or lungs, it can be fatal. Radiation therapy can be effective at decreasing the tumors, but no cure is available. Lymphomas are also more common in AIDS patients. Although HIV is not detected in the malignant cells, it is thought that the virus causes certain growth stimulators of cell proliferation that lead to malignancy.

HIV is detected in the central nervous system, causing an AIDS dementia that can be quite severe. In this case, the virus is causing the disease directly instead of indirectly through an opportunistic infection or cancer. (The same mechanism occurs in the lungs and impairs oxygenation of the blood.) Several opportunistic infections and cancers also affect the nervous system and can lead to death.

The treatment approach to AIDS is twofold. First, two drugs are available that attack the virus and prevent replication in the helper T-cells. They are azidothymidine (AZT) and dideoxyinosine (ddI). Both are recommended for person with HIV infection and ARC when the helper T-cell count falls below 500 cells per milliliter and in all persons who have AIDS. (When the helper T-cell count falls below 200 cells/milliliter, the risk of infection and death are increased.) These drugs are effective in preventing the progression to AIDS and in decreasing the number of opportunistic infections in persons with AIDS, thereby prolonging survival. Side effects are common with these drugs, and sometimes combining the two in lower doses may be more tolerable. Since these drugs can help those with HIV infection before AIDS develops, testing for HIV should not be delayed in high-risk persons. Other drugs with the same actions are being tested and may be available soon.

The second approach is treating opportunistic infections once they occur. New antibiotics have been developed, and new combinations of established drugs have been given to treat these infections. The doses of drugs needed are usually greater in AIDS patients, and antibiotics must often be continued over a long, perhaps indefinite, period. At present, there is no vaccine for HIV, but research is very active in this field.

Prevention is the best defense against AIDS. Blood products are carefully tested for HIV antibodies, and persons at high risk for HIV infection are not to donate blood. Needle sharing is still a problem in large inner cities, and little progress has been made in stopping transmission from this source. "Safe sex" is a phrase that has gained popularity since the advent of AIDS. It must be emphasized that risk cannot be absolutely eliminated when engaging in sex with a partner, no matter what precautions are taken. Latex condoms with spermicide are the best line of defense against the spread of sexually transmitted diseases, including AIDS. Attempting to assess someone's risk factors before engaging in sex is foolish, especially with HIV infections on the rise in the heterosexual population. With such high risks, it is always best to use condoms with any sexual activity.

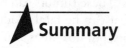 **Summary**

The AIDS epidemic has increased the public awareness and knowledge about the immune system. This devastating disease is caused by a virus transmitted by sexual and blood contact. It slowly destroys the body's cellular defense system against a variety of opportunistic diseases. Public education on the prevention of disease spread has been effective in some sectors, yet many persons are not consistently protecting themselves from this deadly virus. Although remarkable advances have been made in the treatment of HIV infection and opportunistic diseases, no cure or vaccine is currently available.

14 Respiratory System

CASE PRESENTATION

When Bill was in grade school, he had asthma. He often had episodes during which he could not catch his breath and had difficulty breathing. He was taken to the doctor's office and the emergency room on occasion when he was extremely short of breath and was wheezing. Strenuous activity and cold temperatures seemed to make his asthma worse. During the winter months, he took medication. When he was in college, his symptoms decreased, and he discontinued his medication.

When Bill reached age 65, he began complaining of increasing shortness of breath with activity. He noticed these symptoms even when he walked to the end of the driveway to get the mail, and he was no longer able to do the yard work. He also had a cough in the morning that was nonproductive (no sputum produced), but denied any fever and otherwise felt well.

When he saw his physician, he did admit to smoking one to two packs of cigarettes a day since the time he had entered college (approximately 70 "pack-years"). He worked primarily in an office and was not exposed to any asbestos that he was aware of.

His physical exam was mostly normal. His lungs were clear, but his chest appeared barrel shaped, with an increased anterior-to-posterior diameter. A chest x-ray was obtained. The physician told Bill that he probably had emphysema and ordered some breathing tests before starting medication.

Despite the medication, Bill's condition worsened and one evening his breathing was so bad that he went to the emergency room. Shortly after arrival, he was placed on a ventilator to support his breathing.

Questions

1. How do asthma and emphysema differ in their etiology and prognosis?
2. Why does emphysema occur in adults exclusively?
3. Can either of these diseases be cured?
4. What other lung diseases are caused by smoking?

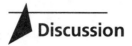

Discussion

Diseases of the lungs and airways are common, perhaps the most common clinical problems. Everyone has suffered from a cold, and asthma among children and emphysema in adults require extensive medical care. A *pulmonologist* is a physician specializing in pulmonary diseases. A chest x-ray is very useful in detecting of some lung diseases (such as pneumonia or certain cancers), but often a CAT scan of the lungs and upper airways provides much more information.

A *bronchoscopy* is a procedure in which a small, flexible, fiber-optic scope is passed into the trachea and into the bronchi. This allows visualization of the airways and the opportunity to obtain a biopsy of the lung parenchyma. This technique is also therapeutic, as mucus plugs in the bronchioles can be removed.

Only a few laboratory tests are useful in the diagnosis and treatment of respiratory diseases. The most information can be obtained from an *arterial blood gas* analysis (ABG). With this study, blood from an artery (usually the brachial or radial artery) is sampled for pH, oxygen, and carbon dioxide. *Hypoxemia* is a condition in which the oxygen content in the blood is abnormally low, indicating poor oxygen delivery to the tissues. Hypoxemia is caused by a host of heart and lung diseases. The immediate treatment for hypoxemia is the administration of supplemental oxygen. When this is done, the amount of oxygen in the inspired air can be increased, to nearly 100% oxygen, so that more oxygen can reach the blood and therefore the tissues. Some persons with chronic, severe lung disease (like emphysema) may be dependent on oxygen just to maintain daily living.

If the hypoxemia is so severe that it cannot be corrected with supplemental oxygen, mechanical ventilatory support is deemed necessary. A *ventilator* is a mechanical support system in which an endotrachial tube (into the trachea through the nose or mouth) is attached to a mechanical pump that delivers a gas mixture to the lungs. The "breaths" are delivered at a certain rate and are intended to coincide with the patient's own respiratory effort. This treatment modality is most effective when used temporarily while the underlying cause of the hypoxia is treated, and then the machine and tube are removed.

Pulmonary function tests (PFTs), often called "breathing tests," are another useful way of measuring respiratory function. Respiratory compliance, airway resistance, and lung capacity and volumes can be measured with the assistance of a spirometer. PFTs are used to diagnose chronic lung diseases and to follow the course of disease progression.

Respiratory Tract Infections

The respiratory tract is vulnerable to infections because it is constantly exposed to airborne *pathogens*. (A pathogen is any agent that causes a disease.) Despite its protective mechanisms (cilia, mucus production, local antibodies), infections are common, especially in the upper respiratory tract. These are called *upper respiratory infections*, or URIs. URIs typically involve the pharynx and have symptoms of a sore throat, fever, cough, and generalized malaise. This is called a *pharyngitis*. Usually, the pathogen is a virus, and the course of the URI is self limited because the body is able to attack and destroy the virus. However, it is possible for bacteria to invade the mucosa already injured by the virus. Bacterial infections are more serious and are best treated with antibiotics. It is not always easy to determine if the infection is caused by a virus or a bacterium, but a cough productive of purulent (pus-like) sputum suggests bacteria as the culprit.

A throat culture is obtained by swabbing the back of the pharynx with a sterile cotton swab and culturing bacterial growth. Viruses are not detected on a throat culture, and there are many bacteria present in the mucosa linings that are not harmful. The best utilization for a throat culture is to diagnose strep throat, which must be treated with antibiotics to prevent complicating kidney or heart diseases.

Laryngitis occurs when the infection involves the vestibular folds and true vocal cords. Hoarseness or loss of voice may result. *Sinusitis* develops when the infection involves the mucosal linings of the sinuses, and *rhinitis* is the inflammation of the nasal mucosa, resulting in a runny nose. Remember, allergies can also cause sinusitis and rhinitis. *Bronchitis*, either viral or bacterial, is the infection of the mucosa of the bronchi and causes a cough. Rarely, it can be detected on a chest x-ray. The treatment for URIs is largely directed at relief of symptoms until the virus runs its course. This includes acetaminophen (Tylenol) or aspirin-like medications for fever and headache and a decongestant and cough suppressant as needed. If antibiotics are prescribed, it is important to complete the entire course (usually seven to ten days) to completely eliminate the bacteria and prevent resistant bacteria strains from developing.

Pneumonia

Pneumonia is a lower respiratory infection of the lung. Pneumonia can be caused by viruses, bacteria, or other infectious agents (recall *pneumocystis carnii* pneumonia in persons with AIDS). A "walking pneumonia," usually caused by a virus or a bacterium-like organism called *mycoplasma*, is less severe and does not require hospitalization for treatment. However, pneumonia caused by bacteria can be quite serious and can be fatal even in this age of antibiotic therapy.

The symptoms of pneumonia include cough, fever, chills, fatigue, and malaise. The involved lung segments are seen on chest x-ray, and an elevated white blood cell count is usually present. The sputum brought up by coughing is cultured to detect the pathogen in most cases, and treatment includes antibiotics (except in viral infections), often given intravenously. As mentioned, mycoplasma pneumonia can be treated with oral antibiotics on an outpatient basis.

"Double pneumonia" is a lay term for bilateral pneumonia. Typically, a bacterial infection is limited to one or two lobules because the infection cannot easily spread between bronchopulmonary segments. An entire lobe of the lung can become infected (lobar pneumonia), but the bacteria rarely spread to the other lung. When this does occur, it is generally quite serious. On the other hand, viral and mycoplasma pneumonias are commonly diffuse infections involving both lungs.

Asthma

Asthma is a common disease, affecting approximately 10% of all children and 5% of all adults. It is usually a disease of childhood, with most of those affected developing symptoms in the first decade of life and a majority of the remainder doing so before the fourth decade. People with asthma experience wheezing, breathing difficulties, and coughing. Those with childhood asthma often experience a relief of symptoms during adulthood, but other people do not develop problems until adulthood. Although the symptoms can be quite bothersome, and at times severe, asthma is rarely fatal and can usually be treated with inhalers and medications.

Asthma is a disease of the airways. The muscle tissues in the bronchial walls contract, fluid and cells accumulate in the walls of the airways, and thick secretions enter the lumens of the airways (Figure 14.1). (These conditions are similar to those affecting the nose in allergies such as hay fever.) The result is a narrowing of the airway lumens and an increase in the work of breathing. The inspiratory phase of breathing is often not affected greatly; rather, it is the inability of air to leave the lungs through narrowed airways that causes respiratory compromise. Air becomes trapped in the lungs after expiration, resulting in hyperinflated lungs and inadequate gas exchange. With treatment, the airways are opened and mucus is removed. No permanent lung damage results.

Allergic asthma is caused by certain substances that trigger these reactions. Seasonal airborne particles, pollution, exercise, infections, and emotional stress can all precipitate an allergic asthma attack. Some people, however, do not have an identifiable cause of their asthma. The reactions in the lungs of these people are the same as in those with allergic asthma. Asthma attacks are intermittent and usually last minutes to hours. Less fre-

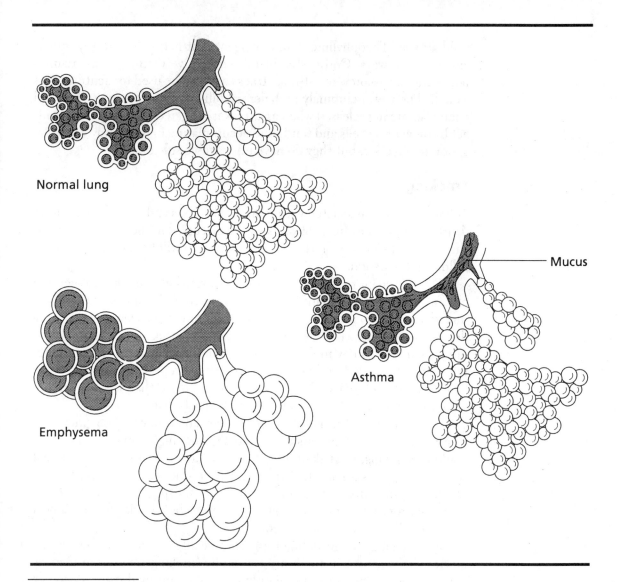

FIGURE 14.1

Histological demonstration of alveoli. The alveolar structure is destroyed in emphysema, resulting in permanent parenchymal damage. Asthma, on the other hand, is caused by reversible swelling of the airways and excess mucus production. The alveolar structure remains intact.

quently, an episode lasts for more than a day. Many asthmatics have long periods without any symptoms or have symptoms only during times of the year when pollen and mold counts are high.

Asthma is treated in many ways. In acute asthma attacks, inhalers containing chemicals with actions similar to those of the sympathetic nervous system are used. These agents dilate the airways so that air movement is easier. These agents can be employed regularly to deter attacks or treat mild attacks. Theophylline is an oral agent that helps clear airway mucus and dilate airways. Corticosteroid inhalers are very effective as maintenance therapy to prevent asthma attacks and can be used for acute attacks as well. The newer chromalyn inhalers stabilize cells in airways so harmful chemicals are not released when an attack is triggered. Oral corticosteroids act by preventing cells and fluid from accumulating in the airway walls and are quite effective, but they do have undesirable side effects.

Smoking

Tobacco abuse is associated with many health risks and leads to premature death. Many of the effects of smoking are discussed in the last chapter, but the effects of smoking on the respiratory system will be mentioned in the following discussion.

The two main risks associated with cigarette smoking are cancer and chronic lung diseases. Nearly 85% of lung cancers and emphysema cases are directly related to smoking, and the total number of cigarettes smoked determines the risk. The greater the number of "pack-years" (the number of packs smoked a day multiplied by the number of years spent smoking) the greater this risk. In other words, if you smoke a pack a day for 40 years, you have 40 pack-years. However, your risk is more than doubled if you smoked two packs a day for 50 years, or 100 pack-years.

Lung cancer is the number one cancer killer among U.S. men and women. The risk of lung cancer is 10 to 25 times higher in smokers. Once you quit smoking, the risk of lung cancer returns to normal over the next seven to ten years. In addition to lung cancer, smoking also causes cancer of the mouth, throat, and esophagus. Cigar and pipe smokers have the same risks for these cancers as cigarette smokers, but the risk of lung cancer and other diseases is not increased.

Emphysema is a very debilitating, chronic disease caused largely by cigarettes. The changes in the lungs caused by smoking are seen in teenage smokers and can progress until emphysema is a limiting disease. However, if one stops smoking before irreversible damage to the lung occurs, the risk of developing emphysema is returned to normal in approximately ten years.

Other common side effects of smoking include an irritating cough, increased mucus production, and nasal congestion. These symptoms resolve shortly after quitting, and overall improved well-being will result.

Chronic Lung Disease

There are two categories of chronic lung diseases, obstructive and restrictive. *Restrictive lung diseases* are the less common. They have many causes (asbestos, radiation, drugs, other diseases) but are not caused by smoking. The primary pulmonary abnormality is the inability to fully inflate the lungs because they are noncompliant, or restricted. Diagnosis is made by chest x-ray and PFTs, but the only treatment is supplemental oxygen and correction of the underlying disease. These diseases are rarely reversible and can be fatal.

Chronic obstructive pulmonary disease (COPD) includes the common disease emphysema. *Emphysema* is a disease in which the alveolar structure breaks down, resulting in the loss of functional lung parenchyma (see Figure 14.1). This loss of parenchyma has two consequences. First, there are fewer alveolus-capillary surfaces for gas exchange. This causes a decrease in blood oxygen. Second, the elastic recoil and structural support of the lungs are destroyed, and the airways collapse, or become obstructed, during expiration. This results is "air trapping" in the lungs because the inspired air cannot be expired through the collapsed airways. Now when the next breath is attempted, the lungs are already filled with air low in oxygen and high in carbon dioxide that was trapped from the last breath.

The symptoms of emphysema are decreased exercise tolerance and shortness of breath. The body reacts to this disease in several ways. 1) The chest cavity expands anteriorly-posteriorly as the lungs become hyperinflated from the air trapping. This can be seen in appearance and on chest x-ray. 2) A greater proportion of the respiratory cycle is spent in expiration to allow more air to escape from the lungs. Also, exhaling against pursed lips will keep the collapsing airways open longer by keeping airway pressure elevated. 3) The resulting hypoxia triggers the production of more red blood cells to increase the oxygen capacity of the blood so that any oxygen reaching the capillaries will be taken into the blood. 4) The central control of breathing changes to one that is driven by the partial pressure of oxygen in the blood instead of the amount of carbon dioxide. When this occurs, giving too much supplemental oxygen can be deleterious because the increased oxygen in the blood will suppress the respiratory center, and respiratory effort will actually decrease.

Treatment of emphysema is largely supportive, as the disease process cannot be cured once alveolar destruction occurs. Supplemental oxygen, inhalers that dilate the airways, corticosteroids (like prednisone), and theophylline appear to relieve symptoms.

Chronic bronchitis is another obstructive lung disease caused by smoking, but the obstruction is not due to alveolar destruction. Rather, large amounts of thick secretions are produced by the airways, and this mucus blocks the airways. Patients have a chronic cough productive of large amounts of sputum every day. The airway obstruction has the same physiological effects as emphysema and is not easily reversible.

Cystic Fibrosis

Cystic fibrosis is a hereditary disease in which the exocrine glands of the body secrete abnormally thick mucus. The two organs most commonly affected are the lungs and the pancreas. In the lungs, the thick secretions plug small airways and can lead to collapse of lung segments. There is also a much higher risk of pneumonia, especially that caused by certain bacteria that are difficult to treat. Respiratory difficulty and recurrent infections are the main symptoms of cystic fibrosis and often lead to the diagnosis of the disease. Intestinal abnormalities and malabsorbtion are also quite common.

The treatments of the pulmonary complications of cystic fibrosis include exercises and treatment to remove the mucus plugs from the lungs. Prompt antibiotic therapy for pneumonia is also important. Persons with cystic fibrosis can now live into their 20s or 30s (the disease was once fatal during childhood), and with improved treatment modalities, many may live to age 50 or more. Genetic counseling is available for families with a history of cystic fibrosis to determine the risk of giving birth to an infant with the disease.

Pneumothorax

A *pneumothorax* is the presence of air in the pleural cavity. This is usually caused by trauma to the chest wall, as in an automobile accident or a knife or gunshot wound. A pneumothorax is also a complication of emphysema because the damaged parenchyma may rupture and allow inspired air to escape into the pleural space. When air enters the pleural space, the pleural linings loose their ability to assist with inflation of the lungs. As more air enters the pleural space, the lung may actually be compressed by the air because there is a limited amount of space in the thoracic cavity. Ventilation is compromised when this occurs, and prompt treatment is required.

Treatment of a pneumothorax involves the evacuation of air from the pleural space. This can be done by inserting a needle through the chest wall and into the pleural space, thus allowing the air to escape through the needle and allowing the lung to reinflate. Once this is accomplished, a *chest tube* is usually placed to provide continuous suction of the air out of the pleural space. A chest tube is about the size of a small finger and is placed between the ribs through a small incision and into the pleural space. It is then connected to suction apparatus that sucks the air out of the pleural cavity. This allows time for healing of the injury, and then the chest tube can be removed.

Lung Cancer

Lung cancer is the leading cause of death due to cancer among U.S. men and women. Nearly 150,000 deaths are caused by lung cancer each year, and the number is increasing among women. The major risk for lung cancer is cigarette smoking. Fortunately, this risk returns to normal 10 to 15 years after stopping.

Lung cancer may be asymptomatic and is sometimes detected incidentally on a chest x-ray or CAT scan obtained for other reasons. Other persons with lung cancer will complain of a persistent cough, shortness of breath, or chest pain. *Hemoptysis* is the coughing of blood and is a symptom of lung cancer, although other diseases may also cause hemoptysis. Once the cancer has spread, symptoms may arise due to the metastasis. For example, if the cancer spreads to the brain, seizures, confusion, and stroke symptoms may occur.

The diagnosis of lung cancer is confirmed by CAT scan or bronchoscopy with a biopsy. Since other diseases can cause a lung mass and different types of lung cancer (there are four) respond better to different treatments, obtaining tissue with a biopsy is critical.

Treatment of lung cancer is largely determined by the size of the tumor and whether it has metastasized. If the tumor is small and confined to the lung, surgical removal of the tumor followed by radiation or chemotherapy may lead to a cure. If surgery is not possible, these two treatments will shrink the tumor and metastases, but a cure is unlikely. In this case, survival at five years is only 10%, and if metastases are present at diagnosis, survival may be only six months.

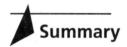

Summary

Respiratory diseases may involve the airways or the lung parenchyma. Most pulmonary diseases lead to impaired gas exchange and the tissues do not receive enough oxygen. This causes symptoms of shortness of breath and fatigue. When an infection or irritant is present in the lungs or airways, a cough occurs, which may be productive of pus-like sputum or even blood.

Respiratory infections are common and can occur in any of the respiratory structures. Most upper airway infections are caused by viruses and do not usually require antibiotic treatment. On the other hand, pneumonia can be fatal, and antibiotic therapy and even hospitalization may be required.

Lung cancer and chronic obstructive pulmonary diseases are largely caused by smoking cigarettes. Asthma is not caused by smoking, although children whose parents smoke have a higher risk of developing the disease. Allergies play a role in asthma, and no permanent lung damage is done with an asthma attack. Asthma and obstructive lung diseases both cause airway obstruction, but the mechanisms by which this occurs are different. Unlike asthma, emphysema results in irreversible damage to the lung parenchyma. Since cigarettes are responsible for 85% of lung cancer and emphysema, avoiding or stopping this dangerous habit will certainly decrease the risk of developing these debilitating, fatal diseases.

15 Digestive System

CASE PRESENTATIONS

Ralph, 37, complained of heartburn. He described the pain as a burning sensation in the midline of his chest. The pain was worse after eating and when he lifted heavy objects. He started taking antacid tablets and had temporary relief of his symptoms, but subsequently he had difficulty falling asleep because of the pain.

Ralph saw his family physician about his symptoms. His doctor asked him about his diet, alcohol consumption, coffee drinking, and smoking. Ralph admitted that he ate fast foods often at lunch and had a large meal late in the evening. He drank five to six cups of coffee each day and usually had a couple of beers in the evening. He had not smoked for four years.

On physical exam, Ralph was moderately overweight and his blood pressure was borderline elevated. Otherwise, his exam was entirely normal, including a test for blood in the stool.

Ralph was told he had heartburn (gastro-esophageal reflux) and was advised to cut back on his coffee and alcohol use and start a low-fat diet, avoiding chocolate. The doctor also recommended an antacid and asked Ralph to call in two weeks if his symptoms persisted.

Ralph's wife, Ruth, also 37, complained of abdominal pain. she felt an intense, dull pain located in the upper center of the abdomen. It was worse before she ate and actually resolved with meals. She started taking some of her husband's antacid tablets and felt better. She had the same dietary habits as her husband, and she smoked cigarettes.

When Ruth saw the doctor, her exam revealed tenderness in the upper abdomen and blood in the stools. She was told she probably had ulcer disease and was given the same advice as Ralph and told she should stop smoking. She was also scheduled for special x-ray studies.

Questions

1. What is heartburn, or gastro-esophageal reflux?
2. How are the symptoms of reflux and ulcer disease different?
3. Why is the treatment of reflux and ulcer disease the same?
4. What causes these two diseases?

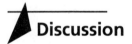

Discussion

Diseases of the digestive system involve either the gastrointestinal (GI) tract or the associated digestive organs. A *gastroenterologist* is a physician specializing in these diseases. The tools a gastroenterologist has available are blood tests, x-ray studies, and endoscopy.

The most useful blood tests are the red cell count and liver function studies. Several GI diseases will result in blood loss from the digestive tract in the stools. If the blood loss occurs over a long period, anemia will result and be detected on a blood test. Liver function studies consist of measuring the amount of liver enzymes in the blood. When there is an abnormality affecting the liver, the amount of enzymes "leaked" into the blood will increase, and the extent of elevation is indicative of the severity of the disease.

An abdominal x-ray shows the amount of gas and feces in the intestines. CAT scans and ultrasound studies are useful for detecting abnormal masses, enlarged organs, and other structural problems. Other specialized studies involve outlining the digestive tract by radio-opaque x-ray solutions to visualize a mass or ulcer.

Endoscopy involves passing a small, flexible, fiber-optic scope into the GI tract to visualize the lining of the esophagus, stomach, duodenum, and colon. To examine the upper GI tract, the endoscope is passed through the mouth and then swallowed. A *colonoscopy* is used to evaluate the lower GI tract (namely, the colon) and is inserted into the rectum and colon. With either procedure, a biopsy can be obtained and the tissue further analyzed to make a diagnosis.

Heartburn

Heartburn is caused by the reflux of stomach contents into the lower esophagus and is called *gastro-esophageal reflux* (GER). GER is caused by relaxed lower esophageal sphincter tone, which allows the acidic gastric contents to enter the esophagus and irritate the esophageal lining. When this occurs, symptoms include a burning sensation in the chest and a bitter taste in the mouth. Sometimes, the gastric contents may reflux back into the mouth. These symptoms typically occur after meals or when lying down or bending over. They resolve gradually over time.

The diagnosis of GER is largely based on symptoms and can be confirmed with x-rays studies and endoscopy. A barium swallow is a special x-ray in which barium (a radio-opaque liquid) is swallowed and then x-rays are taken to detect reflux of barium into the esophagus. Endoscopy is performed to visualize damage in the esophagus caused by chronic reflux and to obtain biopsies of inflamed tissue or esophageal ulcers. Endoscopy is also used to document healing of esophageal disease once the GER has been treated.

Avoiding certain substances that relax the lower esophageal sphincter such as fatty foods, chocolate, alcohol, and nicotine can decrease the amount of reflux. Weight loss, eating smaller meals, avoiding lying down after eating, and sleeping with the head of the bed elevated will favor keeping gastric contents in the stomach. Avoiding esophageal irritants such as coffee and citrus juices will also decrease symptoms.

Medication may be needed if these changes in lifestyle do not alleviate symptoms. The aim of medical treatment is to decrease the amount of acid in the gastric contents so that less irritation is produced with reflux. Antacids neutralize the hydrochloric acid produced by the stomach, and certain histamine blockers decrease the amount of acid produced by the parietal cells. Other medications leave a protective coating on the damaged esophagus, increase sphincter tone, or increase gastric emptying. Frequently, a combination of medications is needed to control symptoms and prevent further esophageal injury.

Peptic Ulcer Disease

An ulcer is a shallow, erosive, open sore caused by some form of injury. In the upper digestive tract, ulcers are caused by an imbalance between digestive elements and the protective mechanisms of the mucosa. When excess acid and pepsin are produced in the stomach, the balance is tipped, and these agents cause irritation of the mucosa, often leading to ulcers. This process is called *peptic ulcer disease*. Nearly 80% of ulcers are in the duodenum, where the acidic stomach contents are emptied. The majority of the others are in the stomach.

Abdominal pain is the most common symptom of peptic ulcer disease. This pain is usually most severe before meals when there is no food in the stomach or duodenum to buffer the acid and pepsin. The pain is located in the upper-middle abdomen and is described as intense, dull, and nagging. Vomiting is also common, and the vomitus may contain either fresh blood or clotted blood that looks like coffee grounds. Bleeding from the ulcers leads to blood loss through the GI tract in the stool. If the bleeding goes on over a long period, anemia will result. In fact, ulcers may be asymptomatic until the symptoms of anemia occur.

The diagnosis of peptic ulcers can be made in two ways. First, an upper GI x-ray study involves swallowing barium, which will outline the lining of the stomach and the proximal small intestine. An ulcer will appear as a punched out area or an irregular area in the mucosal lining. Second, an endoscopy is performed by passing a small fiber-optic tube through the mouth to visualize the digestive tract. Biopsies are also obtained to look for cancer or an infectious cause of the ulcer disease. Blood tests are useful only to determine the presence of anemia.

As with gastro-esophageal reflux, behavioral habits are major risk factors for developing peptic ulcer disease. Smoking is the greatest risk factor for developing ulcers and it also delays their healing. Even smoking ten cigarettes a day can increase your risk for peptic ulcer disease. Caffeine, emotional and physical stress, and alcohol also contribute to ulcer formation. Interestingly, even decaffeinated coffee stimulates acid secretion by the stomach. Aspirin and aspirin-like medications can cause peptic ulcer disease, especially in the elderly population taking these medications for arthritis pain. Men are more apt to develop this disease, and there appear to be genetic influences as well.

The treatments of peptic ulcers are similar to the treatment of gastro-esophageal reflux, with the common goal of decreasing the amount of acid produced by the stomach. Antacid, histamine blockers, and agents that coat the mucosal lining are used in some combination to decease symptoms and promote ulcer healing. Needless to say, lifestyle changes are also very important in the prevention and treatment of peptic ulcer disease.

Diarrhea

Diarrhea is defined as the increased frequency or amount of feces, which are usually watery. This is a very common symptom with many different causes. The most common cause of diarrhea is *gastroenteritis*, an intestinal infection by either bacteria or viruses. Bacterial infections are most common and cause diarrhea by directly attacking the mucosa or by producing a toxin the affects the mucosa. Bacterial infections usually occur by ingesting contaminated food, whereas viral infections are spread by person-to-person contact. Other causes of diarrhea are alcohol, certain drugs, intestinal or colon diseases, and lactose intolerance. In lactose intolerance, the enzyme lactase is lacking in the intestine, and the carbohydrate lactose cannot be digested. The undigested carbohydrate "pulls" water along with it through the gut, causing diarrhea. Avoiding foods containing lactose (like milk) prevents symptoms.

Other symptoms may be present with diarrhea. Nausea, vomiting, and abdominal cramps are common coexisting symptoms. Fever, headache, light headedness, and malaise occur more commonly with gastroenteritis. When there is blood present in the diarrhea, the disease is more serious, and endoscopy should be performed to secure the diagnosis.

The natural course of gastroenteritis is self-limited in most cases, usually lasting from one to five days. Blood tests and stool samples are not needed in this situation, but if fever, diarrhea, and bloody stools persist for two to three days, these should be done along with endoscopy. The blood test will show the degree of blood loss (anemia will result), and the white cell count will be elevated in serious infections or diseases. Stool sample analysis for white blood cells and a culture to identify the infectious agents are very useful in directing therapy.

The treatment of gastroenteritis is fluid replacement until the symptoms resolve. If diarrhea is severe and accompanied by vomiting, intravenous fluid may be required to prevent dehydration. Immodium is a drug that decreases intestinal motility, thereby decreasing the frequency of defecation. This medication should be used sparingly, as constipation may result if too much is taken. Certain bacterial and protozoan infections (giardiasis, for example) require antibiotics to rid the intestine of the organisms. Recovery is complete in all cases once the infection resolves, but resistance to antibiotics occasionally develops, so that repeat infections are possible.

Appendicitis

The appendix is a small organ that creates a lot of attention when it becomes infected. Infection of the appendix is called *appendicitis* and results when the normal gut bacteria invade the appendix mucosa. This occurs when feces block the appendix, thereby trapping bacteria in the appendix, or when the appendix mucosa is damaged. If the infection progresses, the appendix is stretched and can rupture, spilling infected contents into the peritoneal cavity. Serious illness occurs when this happens, so once an appendicitis is diagnosed, the treatment is surgical removal before rupture occurs. Removal of the appendix is called an *appendectomy*.

Abdominal pain is the primary symptom of an appendicitis. This pain is dull at first, starting near the umbilicus. Then it becomes more severe and shifts to the lower right portion of the abdomen. Loss of appetite, nausea, and vomiting may also be present. On exam, the abdomen is very tender and bowel sounds may be absent. The white blood cell count is usually elevated, but x-rays are not useful in making the diagnosis. Once the diagnosis is suspected, an appendectomy should be done to prevent rupture. Recovery is 100%, and the GI system functions normally without the appendix.

Colon Cancer

Colon cancer is the most common cancer of the GI tract. It is a disease of developed countries with diets rich in animal fats and low in dietary fiber. (Refer to the last chapter for the effects of diet on cancer.) There is a minor hereditary risk factor for developing colon cancer, and a discrete cause of colon cancer has not been determined.

Colon cancer arises in the lining of colon and grows into the lumen. It may spread to surrounding tissues, or it may metastasize to the lymph nodes, liver, or lung. If it is diagnosed when still confined to the colon, surgical removal of the cancerous segment of the colon is curative. If however, the cancer has spread out of the colon, a cure is unlikely, and the survival at five years is only 20% with surgery and chemotherapy.

Colon cancer may be asymptomatic for a long period. When the cancer is large enough, it may cause constipation or a decrease in stool caliber. It may go undetected until it completely blocks the colon, causing fecal obstruction, or diarrhea may occur. Colon cancers typically bleed into the colon, and this may cause the stools to become black in appearance. Blood loss in the stool can also be detected by rectal examination and by sampling the stool for occult blood. If blood loss has occurred over a long period, anemia may result, which is detected on a blood test.

Since early detection can lead to surgical resection and cure, any person with symptoms or blood in the stool should have further evaluation with colonoscopy or a barium enema. If a mass is present in the colon, the barium will outline the tumor on an x-ray. With colonoscopy, the tumor can be biopsied to obtain diagnosis, and any precancerous masses can be removed. Routine endoscopy after the age of 50 and yearly testing for blood in the stool are recommended for early detection of asymptomatic colon cancer.

Gallstones

Gallstones are a common problem, affecting 20% of women and 8% of men in the United States over the age of 40. Factors that increase the risk of gallstone formation include obesity, high-fat and high-cholesterol diets, and liver malfunction. The environment of the gallbladder is conducive to gallstone formation when the amount of cholesterol in bile overwhelms the ability of the bile salts (which surround fats and fat-like substances) to prevent cholesterol crystals from forming. If a small crystal forms, it may grow, eventually forming a gallstone.

Some people have gallstones that go unnoticed for years, but in others the stones block the cystic duct or common bile duct (Figure 15.1). Pain in the upper right abdomen is common following meals in people with gallstones and may last for hours. Nausea and vomiting may occur, and if the blockage persists, a serious infection may develop. A decreased intake of fat and cholesterol may alleviate these symptoms, but other treatment is frequently required.

Surgery is often performed in individuals with bothersome gallstones. It is vital in some cases of prolonged obstruction or infection. After removal of the stone-containing gallbladder, bile flows from the hepatic ducts into the common bile duct. The formation of stones is much less likely, although it may still occur under certain circumstances. More recently,

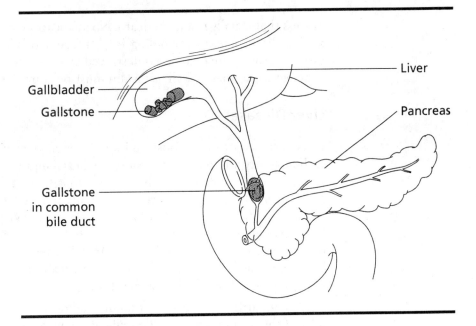

FIGURE 15.1
Gallstones are shown in the gallbladder. Bile flow becomes obstructed if a stone lodges in the common bile duct.

medications have been developed that act to alter the ratio of cholesterol to bile salts in bile, "dissolving" the gallstones. Shock waves have been explored as a method for breaking up gallstones. Although this method has been quite successful in treating kidney stones, it does not appear to be as effective in treating gallstones.

Pancreatitis

Inflammation of the pancreas, *pancreatitis*, is a serious condition. Alcohol and gallstones can contribute to the development of pancreatitis. Alcohol has a direct toxic effect on the pancreas, and gallstones cause damage by blocking the common bile duct, which in most persons fuses with the pancreatic duct. Blockage of the common bile duct thus causes pancreatic juice to back up into the pancreas. Pancreatitis produces severe upper abdominal pain, nausea, vomiting, and loss of appetite. In addition to these symptoms, the elevation of certain pancreatic enzymes in the blood leads to the diagnosis of pancreatitis.

Amylase and lipase are pancreatic enzymes important in the digestion of carbohydrates and fats, respectively. When the pancreas is damaged, these enzymes may leak into the blood instead of emptying into the duodenum. If the pancreatic damage is severe enough, these enzymes, other enzymes, and bicarbonate ions may escape into the abdominal cavity, a process that usually results in death. No medications cure pancreatitis, but resting the pancreas by avoiding food intake allows it to recover. In rare instances the entire pancreas is destroyed by pancreatitis. In these patients pancreatic enzymes as well as insulin must be administered.

Liver Disease

Liver disease is caused most commonly by alcohol or hepatitis viruses. Although very different agents cause the initial injuries to the liver in these cases, the end result is often the same: *cirrhosis,* or hardening and scarring of the liver. The liver has a remarkable ability to regenerate after injury and can even replace a portion that has been removed. With severe, long-term hepatitis caused by viruses or chronic alcohol abuse, however, the liver may become irreversibly damaged. Unfortunately, there is no good way to treat liver failure, although recent advances toward an "artificial liver" may offer some hope short of liver transplantation.

When cirrhosis occurs, liver failure and death may result, because the roles of the liver in digestion, detoxification, metabolism, and protein synthesis are crucial. Several abnormalities accompany liver failure. *Jaundice* is a yellowish coloring of the skin that results when bilirubin levels become high. Bilirubin is a product of hemoglobin breakdown. The liver is responsible for processing this bilirubin; if it is unable to do so, bilirubin accumulates in the body. (Jaundice does not always indicate liver failure.) Another consequence of liver failure is that toxins that the damaged liver cannot degrade accumulate, and the resulting effects on central nervous system function can result in coma. *Ascites,* another complication of liver failure, is the accumulation of fluid in the peritoneal cavity. In this condition, an increased liver blood pressure causes fluid to leak into the peritoneal cavity. Several gallons of fluid may accumulate in this way, and it must often be removed by inserting a needle into the peritoneal cavity. Another consequence of liver failure is kidney damage, which appears to result from the deranged metabolism that accompanies a failed liver. Also, lipid digestion is often impaired. A final consequence of liver failure is decreased levels of key plasma proteins, especially the clotting factors. (Most plasma proteins are synthesized by the liver.) Life-threatening bleeding may occur when levels of clotting factors are low.

Two basic types of viral hepatitis exist, and they are transmitted differently. *Hepatitis A* is transmitted via the digestive tract and contamination of food or water. Hepatitis A usually lasts for only a short time. Fever, abdominal pain, diarrhea, and jaundice are common. The infection, however, is typically destroyed by the body's defenses, and serious complications do not occur. *Hepatitis B* and *hepatitis C* are transmitted by blood, sexual contacts, and body secretions. This type of infection is more serious and can have a long course. Liver failure may result from these blood-borne hepatitis infections. Most cases are contracted sexually or through unsterile intravenous drug needles. Often, medical personnel and certain other groups are vaccinated against hepatitis B.

The connections between alcohol and liver disease warrant further consideration. All forms of alcohol have direct toxic effects on the liver. To a certain degree, the damage can be reversed if alcohol consumption stops. If cirrhosis develops, however, permanent damage has been done. Some 10% to 20% of all alcoholics develop cirrhosis, and 50% show some indication of liver disease. Alcohol is not the only factor contributing to the development of liver disease; genetics, sex, and nutritional factors all seem to play a role. The amount of alcohol that is considered "safe" for the liver is debatable. Even "socially accepted" amounts of alcohol consumed daily over many years probably affect the liver.

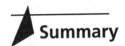

Summary

Diseases of the digestive system can be thought of in three categories: 1) diseases of the upper GI tract (gastroesophageal reflux, peptic ulcer disease), 2) those of the lower GI tract (diarrhea, colon cancer), and 3) diseases of the digestive organs (liver, pancreas and gallbladder disease). Most of these diseases are treated medically with resolution of symptoms. Surgical treatment of some diseases results in a cure of the disease, often by removal of the affected organ or cancer.

Behavioral habits are important in the prevention and treatment of many GI problems. Alcohol use can lead to gastro-esophageal reflux and peptic ulcer disease, both of which improve once drinking is stopped. Liver disease is also caused by alcohol abuse. However, the liver damage is often irreversible and can lead to premature death. Caffeine, smoking, and diets rich in fatty foods also contribute to upper GI diseases.

Colon cancer is potentially curable if detected and treated in early stages. Routine testing for blood in the stool and screening endoscopy after age 50 years are important procedures for decreasing mortality from this cancer.

16 Urinary System

CASE PRESENTATION

Mrs. Smith, at 71, had no chronic medical problems. One day she noticed a red tinge in her urine. She had no pain with urination, but a few hours later she developed a sharp pain in her right flank that radiated around to her right groin. She did not have a fever but did start vomiting. The next time she urinated, her urine was clearly bloody, and her pain was increasing in intensity.

She recalled the previous spring she had a urinary tract infection and her urine was a bit bloody. She also had a great deal of pain when she urinated and a low-grade fever. Her doctor checked a urine sample and prescribed an antibiotic. Within a day she felt better.

Over the next hour, her pain became so severe that she called her doctor, who examined her and admitted her to the hospital. Her physical exam was normal except that she was very tender when the doctor jarred her right flank with his fist. A urine sample revealed blood but no evidence of infection. Her blood work was normal. An abdominal x-ray and special x-ray study confirmed the diagnosis of a kidney stone.

In the hospital, Mrs. Smith was given pain medications and intravenous fluids. Each urine sample was collected and strained until the stone was passed. When this happened, her pain resolved, and so did the bloody urine.

Questions

1. How are kidney stones formed?
2. Why do kidney stones and urinary tract infections both cause blood in the urine?
3. Are all kidney diseases painful?
4. What is dialysis?

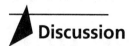

Discussion

Diseases of the urinary system mainly involve the kidneys and bladder. The male prostate gland can become enlarged and cause urinary symptoms, and many men are treated for this problem. An *urologist* is a surgeon specializing in these disorders, and a *nephrologist* is an internist concerned with renal diseases. One way to distinguish the two specialists is that the urologist is concerned with structural abnormalities and the nephrologist with functional problems affecting this system.

The symptoms of urinary tract diseases include *hematuria* (blood in the urine), *dysuria* (painful urination), *frequency* (urinating often), *hesitancy* (difficulty starting the stream), and *incontinence* (inability to control the flow of urine). Many kidney diseases are asymptomatic, like the damage done by hypertension and diabetes, and close evaluation of persons with these risk factors is required to detect kidney damage.

Blood studies are very useful in the diagnosis of urinary tract diseases. An elevated white cell count suggests infection, and anemia results from long-standing kidney disease. The blood also contains waste products, urea and creatinine, that are eliminated by the kidneys. When the kidneys are not functioning properly, these chemicals are not cleared from the blood, and the levels increase. Following these levels indicates the status of the kidney disease. The *urine analysis* (UA) involves testing for certain elements in the urine and examining the urine under a microscope for cells.

The kidneys and bladder can be "visualized" with ultrasound waves to determine size and density. An *intravenous pyelogram* (IVP) is a specialized x-ray study in which a radio-opaque x-ray solution is injected intravenously. As the solution is cleared by the kidneys, it becomes concentrated in the collecting system and bladder. At this point, x-rays can be taken of the outlined collecting system. *Cycstoscopy* is the insertion of a small fiber-optic scope through the urethra to allow visualization of the bladder and ureters.

A *Foley catheter* is a rubber, flexible tube that is inserted through the urethra into the bladder to drain urine. The urine is collected in a bag, and the amount can be measured. A Foley catheter is used in hospitalized patients who are too ill to get out of bed to urinate and those undergoing surgery. Once physical activity increases, the catheter is removed without residual injury.

Kidney Stones

Kidney stones affect young adults as well as the elderly. They are caused by the precipitation of chemicals in the urine and usually form in the renal pelvis. The stone causes irritation when it leaves the pelvis and enters the ureter and continues to do so until it enters the bladder. Most small stones will pass through the ureter on their own, but they rarely do so when the size approaches one-half inch.

The most common symptom of kidney stones is pain. This pain is usually intermittent and starts in the flank on the side of the stone. The pain is described as intense, dull, and throbbing. As the stone descends, so does the pain, and it may become a lower abdominal pain. Hematuria is often present, and nausea and vomiting can occur. Dysuria is not associated with kidney stones, and if it is present, an infection in the kidney must be considered.

The diagnosis of a kidney stone is made by visualizing the stone in the urinary tract. Calcium stones, the most common, can be seen on a regular abdominal x-ray if they are large enough. If the stone cannot be seen, an IVP is performed to localize the stone. The UA may show blood, but there is no evidence of infection, and blood work is normal.

Treatment of kidney stones includes aggressive hydration to "flush" the stone through, pain medication, and removal of the stone if needed. As mentioned above, small stones have a good chance of passing on their own. If the stone is large, surgical removal or lithotripsy is required (Figure 16.1). *Lithotripsy* is the use of shock waves to break the stone into smaller pieces that will pass through the tract. How the treatment is delivered depends on how large the stone is and whether vomiting is present. If the person is able

---

FIGURE 16.1
Surgical removal of a kidney stone. With this percutaneous (through the skin) technique, the kidney stone can be visualized in the ureter. The stone can be clasped by the "basket" and removed.

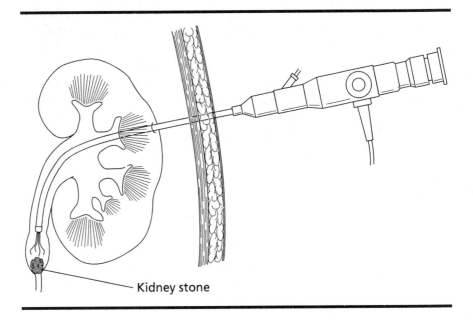

Kidney stone

to drink lots of fluids and keep pain medication down without vomiting, outpatient therapy is effective. However, sometimes hospitalization is needed to administer intravenous fluids and pain control until the stone passes.

It is important to obtain the stone once it passes in the urine to analyze its content. Some types of stones are associated with certain diseases. These and a few other types of stones can be prevented from forming in the future.

Urinary Tract Infections

Urinary tract infections (UTIs) are more common in women than men. Most women will have at least one UTI, and some will be plagued by recurrent infections. The most common site of infection is the bladder. Kidney infections are rare and extremely serious, often requiring hospitalization for intravenous antibiotics. Infections enter the bladder through a women's short urethra. These organisms are generally introduced by wiping with toilet paper after defecation or during sexual intercourse. The risk of infection is increased by dehydration, as there is less urine to flush out the bacteria. UTIs can be prevented by wiping from anterior to posterior and by voiding immediately after intercourse.

Dysuria is the most common symptom. Frequency, hesitancy, and urgency may also be present. Hematuria is common, and the urine may appear cloudy due the number of white blood cells present. Lower abdominal pain (above the pubic bone) may be present and often increases with urination. Fever and aches are less common and may indicate the presence of a kidney infection.

The diagnosis of UTI is made by urine analysis and culture. The UA will show many white blood cells, bacteria, and blood. The culture will identify the organism causing the infection and indicate which antibiotics are effective for treatment.

Treatment is usually by oral antibiotics. Some infections can be treated with a single dose of therapy, but others may require hospitalization for intravenous antibiotics. If the dysuria and abdominal pain are severe, oral medications that become concentrated in the urine can be given for pain relief. Taking certain precautions, as mentioned above, and staying well hydrated will decrease the risk of recurrent infections.

Kidney Cancer

Renal cell carcinomas arise from the cells of the renal tubules and can become very large before they are recognized. Most persons with renal cancer have blood in the urine (hematuria), but this blood is often not visible to the unaided eye and is detected only with the use of a microscope. People with renal cancer may express vague complaints, but rarely are the symptoms specific enough to arouse suspicion of malignancy.

Kidney cancer patients may secrete excessive amounts of the renal hormone erythropoietin. Because this hormone stimulates red blood cell formation, kidney cancer may be accompanied by an increased number of red cells. Excessive renin secretion may occur in kidney cancer as well, leading to hypertension that is secondary to the cancer.

Kidney cancers tend to metastasize to unusual locations. Although renal cancer commonly spreads to the lungs, lymph nodes, liver, and brain, it can spread to virtually any body region, including the eyes and reproductive organs. A second unusual feature of renal cancer is that it exhibits a variety of growth patterns. Some renal tumors show very slow, unnoticed growth over many years. Others exhibit very rapid, sudden growth accompanied by metastasis. The basic aspect of the treatment for renal cell carcinoma is the removal of the affected kidney, and survival rates depend on how widespread the disease is at the time of diagnosis.

Wilm's tumor is a type of kidney cancer that is very different from renal cell carcinoma. Wilm's tumor is a common cancer in children and is seen most often between the ages of 1 and 4 years. This variety of cancer has some bizarre characteristics. For example, it is composed of many different tissue types, including bone, muscle, epithelium, cartilage, and others. The tumor is usually discovered as a large, painful mass in the abdomen, and in many individuals the cancer has spread to the lungs by the time the diagnosis is made. Since the 1960s, advances in surgery, chemotherapy, and radiation therapy have dramatically improved the chances of survival for Wilm's tumor patients.

Dialysis

Dialysis is the separation of molecules based on size and is used in the artificial kidney. An artificial kidney is similar to the thin descending limb of the nephron where molecules travel out of the tubule, down concentration gradients, and into the surrounding fluid outside the tubule. With *hemodialysis* (dialysis of the blood), the arterial blood is pumped through a tube into the dialysis machine. Here it enters a series of very small "capillary" tubes made of a semiperimeable cellophane membrane. This membrane allows molecules smaller than plasma proteins to traverse freely. The semipermeable capillary tubes are surrounded by a fluid called the dialysate. This fluid is poured into the dialysis machine for each dialysis session. The concentration of electrolytes and other molecules in the dialysate will determine whether blood components will diffuse out of the blood, down their concentration gradients, and into the dialysate. Likewise, if the concentration of molecules in the dialysate is the same as in the blood, there is no gradient, and the molecules remain in the blood. Water may also be eliminated by using a hyperosmolar dialysate solution composed of molecules too large to diffuse across the membrane. Through this process, the work of the kidney is accomplished, and important plasma proteins and cells are trapped in the blood. The "cleansed" blood is returned to the body through a tube that enters the vein. (Ten to 15 hours of hemodialysis per week is required to restore normal blood composition. This is usually accomplished in hospitals or clinics, as hemodialysis machines are very expensive and require technical expertise.)

Another option is to use a naturally occurring semipermeable membrane in the body to carry out dialysis. This can be accomplished utilizing the capillaries in the omentum of the abdominal cavity. Instead of removing blood from the body for dialysis, dialysate fluid is introduced into the peritoneal cavity through a small, permanently placed tube. Now dialysis occurs as the blood circulates through these omental capillaries. When the dialysis is complete, the dialysate is removed along with the dialyzed molecules.

The kidneys have a huge functional reserve, and adequate function can occur with only 20% to 30% of the kidney working properly. This allows a person to survive when one kidney is removed because of disease or for organ donation. The most common causes of kidney failure leading to dialysis are diabetes, hypertension, and primary diseases of the nephrons.

Kidney Transplantation

Kidney transplantation has allowed many persons with kidney failure freedom from dialysis. The success rate after transplantation depends on the immunologic response of the recipient in developing host versus graft rejection. If the kidney is rejected by the body, dialysis once again is required until another donor kidney becomes available. In other words, it is possible to have more than one kidney transplant if one fails. With newer drugs to suppress the immune system, the success rate of transplantation from a family member is 90%. If an unrelated donor kidney (which has been immunologically matched to decrease risk of rejection) is transplanted, the success rate is approximately 80%. Unfortunately, many eligible dialysis patients are still waiting for transplantation due to the shortage of donor organs.

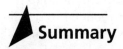 **Summary**

Diseases of the urinary tract may be transient or may result in permanent damage. If the injury destroys 70% to 80% of the kidney function, renal failure occurs, requiring dialysis or kidney transplantation. Several diseases of the urinary system produce symptoms. These diseases are generally transient and cause no permanent damage. On the other hand, diseases that cause irreversible damage, such as diabetes, hypertension, and intrinsic kidney diseases, are asymptomatic.

17 Reproductive System

CASE PRESENTATION

Sandra, 60, saw her gynecologist for her yearly pelvic exam and Pap smear. She did not have any chronic health problems, was active and feeling well, and was taking a calcium supplement to help prevent osteoporosis. Sandra delivered two children, at age 23 and 25 years. She started menopause when she was 48 years old and has not had any menstrual bleeding since that time.

When she was in her 30s, she had an ovarian cyst the size of a table tennis ball. She became aware of the cyst because she had abdominal pain and cramping in the middle of her menstrual cycle when she ovulated. The cyst was palpated and diagnosed on pelvic exam.

On pelvic exam at age 60, an ovarian mass was felt. The gynecologist explained to Sandra that it was very abnormal to have an ovarian mass after menopause. She ordered a CAT scan to better define the mass. The CAT scan showed the mass and there was evidence of enlarged pelvic lymph nodes. This was consistent with the diagnosis of ovarian cancer, and Sandra underwent surgery to have the cancer removed.

Questions

1. Why are benign ovarian cysts extremely uncommon after menopause?

2. What is the prognosis for ovarian cancer?

3. How are yearly pelvic exams and Pap smears helpful?

4. What cancers arise in the male reproductive organs?

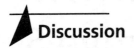

Discussion

Both men and women are plagued by disorders of the reproductive system. In men, the prostate gland is the most bothersome. With age, this gland may enlarge or develop cancer. When this occurs, it may impinge on the ureter, leading to symptoms of urinary hesitancy or frequency. If it is very enlarged, total obstruction of urine flow may occur. A urologist treats prostate disorders in one of two ways. First, a transurethral resection involves placing a catheter in the urethra and utilizing a rotary blade device to cut the prostate. If this is unsuccessful or if cancer is present, the prostate gland is removed by surgery.

A *gynecologist* is a physician specializing in the female reproductive system. Many gynecologists are also *obstetricians* (physicians who deliver babies), but in recent years some gynecologists have given up delivering babies due to malpractice insurance premiums and risk of litigation. A pelvic exam involves the visual inspection of the vulva, insertion of a speculum into the vagina to visualize the vaginal walls and cervix, obtaining samples from the vaginal walls and cervix for microscopic examination, and finally, a bimanual exam. With the bimanual exam, two fingers are inserted into the vagina and the other hand palpates the lower abdomen to feel the uterus and ovaries between the two hands. A Pap smear is the microscopic examination of a sample scraped or brushed from the cervix and vagina. This technique is used to detect early forms of cervical cancer before the lesions become visible to the eye.

Colposcopy is the visualization of the cervix through a specialized microscope during a pelvic examination. This technique can be used to obtain biopsies of any abnormal-appearing area and even treatment of lesions by freezing them (cryotherapy) or via laser. *Laproscopy* employs a fiber-optic tube to visualize and treat lesions in the pelvic cavity. The tube is usually inserted into the abdominal cavity through a tiny incision by the umbilicus. Laproscopy has spared many women exploratory surgery for gynecological problems.

Symptoms Related to the Menstrual Cycle

Menstrual irregularities are common problems. A few of these symptoms will be discussed below. *Dysmenorrhea* is the term for painful menses, commonly thought of as menstrual cramps. Fatigue, headache, and backache may occur in addition to the lower abdominal cramping sensation. Diarrhea, nausea, and vomiting may be so severe as to require hospitalization for intravenous hydration and pain control. Dysmenorrhea is caused by forceful uterine contractions, decreased blood flow to the uterus, and excessive amounts of prostaglandins (which contribute to pain perception). Treatment options for dysmenorrhea include medications that inhibit prostaglandin synthesis like ibuprofen (Motrin, Advil, Nuprin) and naproxen (Anaprox or Naprosyn). If symptoms are so severe as to limit daily activity, birth control medications (estrogen and progesterone) should be considered. This form of treatment is optimal for women who also desire birth control. Women who exercise tend to suffer less from dysmenorrhea, probably because exercise decreases prostaglandins and increases the natural painkillers known as endorphins.

Amenorrhea is the lack of menstrual bleeding. There are several causes of amenorrhea, including structural abnormalities with the reproductive tract, genetic disorders, cancers, and dysfunction of the nervous system. Certain lifestyle habits such as vigorous exercise, excessive weight loss, extreme obesity, severe mental stress, and certain drugs (tranquilizers, opiates, alcohol, and estrogen) may cause amenorrhea. Any woman without menses (without a known cause such as menopause or pregnancy) should see a physician to determine the underlying cause.

Mittelschmerz is a pain or sensation in the lower abdomen, usually occurring at midcycle, indicating rupture of one of the ovarian follicles. This pain may be quite severe if there is rupture of an ovarian cyst and the cyst contents leak into the peritoneum. Ovarian cysts may be asymptomatic and may be detected only on routine pelvic exam. Cysts can become quite large(up to grapefruit size) but typically are less than 2 inches in diameter. Diagnosis can be confirmed by ultrasound, and the cysts can be suppressed by hormone therapy (usually with birth control pills). Some large cysts may require surgical removal of the ovary.

Premenstrual syndrome (PMS) is a collection of emotional, psychological, and physical symptoms that occur during the luteal phase of the menstrual cycle and resolve with the onset of menses. Emotional symptoms include mood swings, depression, crying, panic attacks, anxiety, hostility, irritability, and violence. These symptoms may occur spontaneously or with very little provocation, and women are frustrated with their lack of control over these symptoms. Physical symptoms are headache, fatigue, dizziness, acne, bloating, and breast tenderness and swelling. The cause of PMS is not clearly understood. Alterations and fluctuations in hormone balance may be responsible for many symptoms. They are mediated, in part, through effects on neurotransmitters. The treatment of PMS is symptomatic relief, and for some women a combination of medication and lifestyle changes is helpful. Vitamin B_{12}, anti-inflamatory medications, exercise, avoiding sugar and caffeine, and medications that influence neurotransmitters are possible treatment methods.

Toxic Shock Syndrome

Toxic shock syndrome became epidemic among young women in the 1980s. It is a disease caused by a bacterial infection that starts in the vagina of menstruating women. Hyperabsorbancy tampons that are left in the vagina for a long period provide a surface on which the bacteria can grow. The bacteria then produce a toxin that causes the symptoms of toxic shock syndrome. The syndrome consists of high fever, a red, peeling rash on the palms and soles of the feet, and hypotension (abnormally low blood pressure). Vomiting, diarrhea, muscle aches, and malaise may also occur. These symptoms come on rapidly after the onset of menses. Diagnosis is made by growing the organisms obtained from the vagina. The total white blood cell count is often elevated. Treatment is antibiotic therapy directed against the offending bacteria. The incidence of toxic shock syndrome has decreased with public education and reduced use of hyperabsorbant tampons.

Symptoms of Menopause

Menopause is the cessation of reproductive function in women. Menopause typically occurs between the ages of 45 and 55 and is characterized by decreased estrogen production and ovarian function. The physiological changes of menopause are discussed in textbooks, and the following discussion will de directed to the symptoms of menopause and their treatment.

Hot flashes are the sudden onset of warmth and redness, followed by shaking and profuse sweating. These episodes may occur at any time of the day or night, may occur several times a day, and may last for several minutes. Hot flashes are caused by sporadic hormonal releases from the pituitary gland. Nearly 50% of women will suffer from them, and 15% may not be able to carry out daily activities because of these symptoms. Estrogen replacement therapy is effective at decreasing or eliminating hot flashes.

Genital and breast atrophy occur with the menopausal decrease in circulating estrogen. Although all the reproductive structures shrink, the changes in the vagina and vulva create symptoms of dryness, itching, tenderness, and painful intercourse. These symptoms can be treated with local lubricants and creams that contain estrogen or with oral estrogen replacement therapy.

Osteoporosis (thinning of the bones) is usually an asymptomatic problem. Unfortunately, spinal-compression fractures or a broken hip or wrists occur all too frequently as a result of osteoporosis. Decrease in bone mass starts before menopause but is accelerated by the lack of estrogen. In addition to weight-bearing exercise and proper diet, estrogen replacement therapy decreases the risk of osteoporosis in postmenopausal women.

Like osteoporosis, the acceleration of postmenopausal atherosclerosis may go unnoticed until chest pain, claudication (pain in the legs when walking), or a heart attack occurs. Controlling other risk factors for this disease (smoking, diabetes, hypertension) and estrogen replacement may decrease the risk of these complications.

It is probably obvious that many women may want to or should take estrogen following menopause. The decision is a personal one that should be made with one's physician. However, with all the potential benefits of estrogen replacement, every woman should consider estrogen as a means of preventing symptoms and debilitating diseases. Women who have had breast cancer should *not* take estrogen, and those who have had blood clots caused by estrogen should avoid estrogen in the future. All other women are potential candidates for estrogen therapy. The only significant risk of estrogen replacement is endometrial cancer, and this risk is significantly reduced when estrogen is combined with progesterone. This combination therapy may cause a return of menses, which many women do not desire. Preliminary studies show that certain combinations may be effective, safe, and do not cause menstrual bleeding. Yearly follow-up with a health-care professional is mandatory for screening for early cancer or other problems.

Impotence

Impotence is the inability to achieve or maintain an erection. It affects 10 to 20 million males in the United States. There are two types of impotence, organic and psychogenic. Organic impotence is caused by a physiological abnormality in the nervous system, blood supply, or hormones that contribute to erection. This is the most common cause of impotence, and it affects men with diabetes mellitus and atherosclerosis. Drugs, including alcohol, marijuana, cocaine, tranquilizers, antihistamines, and many blood pressure medications, can cause impotence. Treatment for organic impotence involves the elimination of any causative medications and treatment of underlying diseases. Even so, 30% to 60% of diabetic men still have impotence, and in these situations, penile implants restore some sexual function.

Psychogenic impotence is due to anxiety about sexual performance, stress, depression, or personal sexual experiences. Psychotherapy or sex therapy may be of benefit once an organic cause of impotence is excluded.

Sexually Transmitted Diseases

Sexually transmitted diseases (STDs) are infections that are spread from one person to another during sexual intercourse. Two viruses are transmitted sexually but cause diseases in nongenital tissues. These are HIV, which causes AIDS, and the hepatitis viruses, which cause a liver disease. Neither disease is curable, and AIDS has been fatal thus far. Hepatitis can also be fatal, but a vaccine is available for the prevention of one type of the disease. Both of these viral illness have been discussed in previous chapters. Other sexually transmitted diseases infect and involve the reproductive organs and are discussed below.

Syphilis is a bacterial disease that causes a raised ulcer (chancre) on the external genitalia. This lesion is painless and occurs ten days to three months following sexual contact with an infected person. A chancre can be from very small to larger than an inch in diameter, and more than one may be present (Figure 17.1). Swollen, painless lymph nodes in the groin are also common. The disease is easily treated with an antibiotic, but if it is left untreated, several serious problems may develop months to years later. These include neurological abnormalities, cardiac dysfunction, skin rashes, arthritis, and immunologic reactions.

Genital herpes has been discussed in an earlier chapter. Unlike syphilis ulcers, the blister-like lesions of herpes are usually multiple and very painful. There are secondary recurrences brought on by stress, illness, and other factors, and no cure is available.

Gonorrhea, which is caused by a bacterium, does not cause external genital lesions. Instead, the urethra (in males), and the fallopian tubes, uterus, and vagina are infected. The symptoms include abdominal pain, vaginal discharge, itching, and dysuria. The disease is spread easily from males to females but not as readily from females to males. Males are largely asymptomatic. Unfortunately, asymptomatic women may have scarring of the fallopian tubes, which causes problems with fertility and pregnancy. Gonorrhea can be treated with antibiotics to prevent these serious complications.

Chlamydia causes symptoms similar to gonorrhea but is two to three times more common. The diagnosis of chlamydial infections relies on the

---

FIGURE 17.1
Sexually transmitted diseases. Herpes causes very painful, blister-like lesions. Syphilis is an open ulcer or sore that does not cause discomfort. Genital warts are also painless, but the rough, raised lesions are quite annoying.

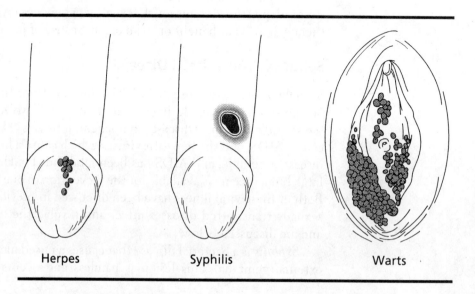

Herpes   Syphilis   Warts

identification of the organism in the penile or vaginal discharge. Chlamydia may also cause reproductive problems and is treated with antibiotics.

Genital warts are STDs caused by viruses. Warts are rough, raised, painless lesions on the external genitalia and can spread to the vagina and cervix (see Figure 17.1). Rarely, vaginal discomfort and itching may occur. Certain types of genital warts are associated with cancerous lesions of the cervix. Treatment involves scraping the warts and "freezing" the base of the lesions or applying topical medication to the warts.

Trichinosis and *gardnerella*, two other STDs, cause vaginal discomfort, itching, and vaginal discharge that is copious and often very odorous. Treatment includes an oral antibiotic (Flagyl), vaginal medicated creams, and vinegar douches for relief of symptoms.

STDs are frequently asymptomatic, so that one may not be aware of the infection and spread it to a partner unknowingly. This infected individual is an asymptomatic carrier of the disease and may infect several sexual partners before the infection is known and treatment given. Once an STD has been diagnosed, the sexual partners also need to be treated to prevent the spread of infection to others. The diagnosis of STDs is by microscopic visualization or culture of the infectious organism. Treatment is then directed at the specific causative organism(s). STDs are more common in persons with multiple sexual partners. Prevention of a majority of STDs can be accomplished by using a latex condom with spermicide. Proper use can decrease the risk of STDs by approximately 90%. Unfortunately, no sex is the only truly safe sex.

Cancers of the Male Reproductive System

The two primary cancers of the male reproductive system are testicular and prostatic cancers. *Testicular cancers* are noticed most often as a painless mass or swelling in a testis. Such a tumor is often inappropriately attributed to an athletic injury. If detected early, before metastasis (spread to another body region), the cancer can nearly always be cured by surgical removal of the affected testis. If the cancer has spread to surrounding lymph nodes, the chance of cure decreases. If it has spread to the thorax, liver, or lungs, aggressive chemotherapy is usually effective only in achieving remissions. Because testicular cancer can be cured if detected early, it is often advised that males (especially those 15 to 34 years old) perform testicular self-examinations, much as many females perform breast self-examinations, and bring to immediate medical attention any mass within or change in the size of a testis.

Prostatic cancer is relatively common in men over 50 years of age and accounts for a large number of cancer deaths. Many tumors that are confined to the prostate gland at the time of diagnosis can be cured by removal of the prostate and the cancerous mass. If the tumor has spread beyond the confines of the prostate gland, the cure rate is very low even with the use of the best treatments available. Prostatic cancer typically spreads to the surrounding lymph nodes, the abdominal cavity, and bones. The presence of cancer in the bones can be extremely painful, and fractures are common. Prostatic cancers may often be detected by rectal examination, in which the posterior surface of the prostate gland is palpated for masses. This examination is especially recommended for males with a family history of prostatic cancer.

Cancers of the Female Reproductive System

The most common cancers of the female reproductive system are breast, cervical, endometrial, and ovarian cancers. *Breast cancer* is the most common of these and is the leading cause of cancer deaths in females. Approximately 11% of all females develop breast cancer during their lifetimes, with the most common time of onset being near menopause. Females with a family history of breast cancer (in a mother, sister, aunt, or grandmother) are at a higher risk of developing breast cancer than others. Also, having had one breast cancer, even if it has been treated successfully, predisposes one to developing another. Obesity, a high dietary fat intake, and the use of alcohol all appear to increase the risk of breast cancer. Other factors that predispose a female to breast cancer include an early onset of menses (before the age of 13 years), having had no children or having had children after the age of 30 years, and late menopause (after the age of 50 years). These last factors suggest a hormonal role in the development of breast cancer, although this idea is unproved.

Over 90% of all cancerous masses in the breasts are first detected by the woman as an incidental finding or by self-examination. With this in mind, most health professionals strongly recommend that women perform self-examinations on their breasts monthly. Annual examinations by a medical professional are also recommended by many physicians, and *mammography* has emerged as an effective screening device for breast cancer. For women at high risk for breast cancer, mammography is recommended starting at 35 or 40 years of age, and for all women over 50 mammography is recommended every year. Mammography, which uses x-rays, is capable of detecting small breast masses that are often missed by self-examinations or medical checkups. Mammography is also used to evaluate further a suspicious mass that has been discovered by examination. The treatment for breast cancer is determined by the amount of metastasis. In cancer confined to the breast, the mass can be removed, and the lymph nodes in the axilla on the affected side can also be removed to look for metastasis. It has become nearly routine for this surgical removal to be followed by some course of chemotherapy, radiation therapy, or hormonal therapy. Unfortunately, breast cancers treated in this fashion may still appear in another body region up to 20 years after treatment. If the cancer has already metastasized at the time of diagnosis, mastectomy is of no benefit, and the prognosis is very poor.

Cervical cancer was the leading cause of cancer deaths in females 50 years ago, but the incidence of deaths from cervical cancer has declined markedly with effective screening for early detection. Cervical cancer is slow growing and can be detected early by routine pelvic examinations and Pap smears. A Pap smear is a method of obtaining a sample of cells from the cervix for microscopic examination. This examination attempts to detect precancerous or suspicious cells. Because the cancer is slow growing, the disease can be treated promptly and effectively if abnormal cells are detected. Precancerous cervical regions may be treated with cryotherapy (freezing), electrocoagulation (electrical burning), local "cone" removal of tissue, laser therapy, or even hysterectomy (removal of the uterus). These precancerous lesions are essentially 100% curable using these methods.

If cervical cancer is undetected and allowed to grow, it invades surrounding structures and may block the urinary bladder and ureters, a situation that can lead to death. Even with surgery, radiation therapy, or both, the five-year survival rate in individuals in whom cervical cancer has invaded surrounding tissues is only about 15%. A high number of sexual partners, an early age of onset of sexual activity, frequent intercourse, a young age at first pregnancy, large numbers of pregnancies, and other factors increase the risk of cervical cancer.

The incidence of *endometrial cancer* is on the rise, especially in women with obesity, diabetes, hypertension, and infertility. This disease is more common after menopause. Endometrial cancer is usually diagnosed when a women seeks medical attention for abnormal uterine bleeding. A large majority of women diagnosed with endometrial cancer have limited disease that can be cured with surgery, which may be followed by radiation therapy. If the disease has spread, the prognosis becomes much worse; thus, health professionals recommended strongly that any abnormal uterine bleeding, especially after menopause, be brought to medical attention.

Ovarian cancers are relatively uncommon, but they account for a disproportionately large number of deaths. This is explained by the fact that they are "silent" (unnoticed) cancers that are typically large and widespread before they are detected. Abdominal pain and swelling are the most likely symptoms to bring ovarian cancer to medical attention. Rarely are these cancers totally removed by surgery, and despite aggressive surgery and chemotherapy, the long-term survival rate for individuals with this disease is low.

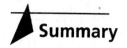

Summary

Diseases of the reproductive system can be functional, structural, or infectious. Early diagnosis of cancers of the male and female reproductive organs can lead to cure. Self-examinations and regular checkups are important for early detection. Prompt treatment of STDs decreases symptoms and spread of the disease, although asymptomatic carriers will continue to cause widespread disease. Use of condoms and monogamous sexual relationships decrease the risk of STDs. Once again, lifestyle changes can make a difference in staying healthy.

18 Pregnancy and Development

CASE PRESENTATIONS

Marie, 27, had two children. She had missed her previous menstrual period and felt she was probably pregnant. A month later she noted some menstrual bleeding and called her physician. She was told that it was not uncommon to have some bleeding in the first trimester of pregnancy but that it might be an early sign of a miscarriage. She came into the office, and her physical examination was normal. Her pregnancy test was positive. Later that evening, Marie developed more bleeding and abdominal cramping. She called her physician and was told to check for small clots, which were indeed present. She was asked to save any tissue she passed that evening. The cramping and bleeding lasted most of the night and then stopped toward morning. She again saw her doctor, and after the tissue was examined was told that she had had a miscarriage.

Mona, 22, had missed her two previous menstrual periods. One day at work she noted some menstrual bleeding and had a dull but significant pain in her lower left abdomen. She began feeling weak and was taken to the emergency room, where she nearly collapsed. Her blood pressure was low, and she was very tender in her lower left abdomen. An obstetrician was called, and Mona had emergency surgery for an ectopic pregnancy.

Questions

1. Is bleeding during pregnancy common?

2. What is a miscarriage?

3. Why is an ectopic pregnancy a medical emergency?

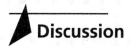

Discussion

Obstetrics is the branch of medicine concerned with pregnancy and childbirth. An *obstetrician* is a physician specializing in the care of women during pregnancy, delivery, and the postpartum period. Many family physicians also care for pregnant women and deliver babies. In addition, they care for the child during early development and deal with the mother's other health-care issues.

The diagnosis of pregnancy is first suspected when the woman misses a menstrual period. The beta-HCG level in the urine of pregnant women is elevated and can be detected by testing. Once a woman learns she is pregnant, medical care should be initiated to ensure a safe pregnancy and healthy development of the fetus. A *sonogram* is an method of visualizing the fetus with the use of sound waves. In this way, an estimation of fetal age and an assessment of fetal growth can be made. Most of the time, the sex of the fetus can also be determined by sonography.

Prevention of pregnancy is an equally important health care issue for many women, men, and couples. There are many options for contraception, each with an accepted efficacy, convenience, and risk for side effects. These will be discussed below.

Ectopic Pregnancy

For the proper development of the fetus, uterine implantation is necessary. However, in 1% of all pregnancies, the fertilized ovum is implanted in a location other than the uterus, most commonly in a fallopian tube. This abnormal site of implantation is called an "ectopic pregnancy" (Figure 18.1). There are two consequences of an ectopic pregnancy. First, the fallopian tubes cannot support fetal growth as the uterus does, and the fetus dies 6 to 14 weeks after fertilization. Second, the fallopian tubes are not as strong as the uterus and rupture when the fetus reaches a certain size. This rupture of the tube can be life threatening to the mother due to excessive bleeding into the abdominal cavity.

Ectopic pregnancies have become more common in recent years, for two reasons. First, more women are becoming sexually active at a younger age and are contracting more sexually transmitted diseases, which may lead to scarring of the fallopian tubes. Second, the use of intrauterine devices (IUDs) for birth control also increases the risk of ectopic pregnancy. Women will complain of abdominal pain and may have abnormal or absent menses. The diagnosis of ectopic pregnancy requires a beta-HCG test, ultrasound study, or laproscopic exam (inserting a "scope into the peritoneal cavity and taking a look). In most cases, surgery is required to stop the bleeding and remove the dead fetus. Recently, experimental use of medi-

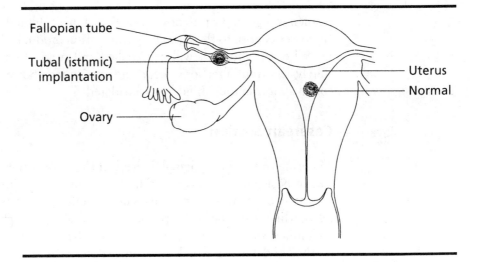

Fallopian tube

Tubal (isthmic)
implantation

Ovary

Uterus

Normal

FIGURE 18.1

Ectopic pregnancy. Normal implementation of the embryo is in the uterus. In an ectopic pregnancy, implantation may occur in a fallopian tube (a tubal pregnancy).

cation has been promising for early treatment of ectopic pregnancy before rupture occurs.

Miscarriage

An *abortion* is the interruption of a pregnancy with the "delivery" of a nonviable fetus. A miscarriage is a spontaneous, natural abortion prior to the time when the fetus can survive outside of the uterus (usually before the 20th week of gestation at a weight of less than a pound). Fifteen percent to 20% of pregnancies spontaneously abort in the first trimester. Although a miscarriage is an unfortunate event for an expectant couple, spontaneous abortion is nature's way of selecting out fetuses that could not survive.

The great majority of miscarriages are caused by genetic defects. Chromosomal abnormalities account for over half of these abortions, and the majority of these are due to autosomal trisomies. An autosomal trisomy is the replication of a chromosome or part of a chromosome so that three copies instead of the usual two are present. The most common trisomy is trisomy 16, which is uniformly lethal before birth. Trisomy 21 is also common, but unlike trisomy 16 it is not lethal, and infants with trisomy 21 have Down's syndrome.

The symptoms of a spontaneous abortion include bleeding followed by a cramping abdominal pain and passage of the conception material. Almost one-quarter of women will have some bleeding during the first half of pregnancy. This is considered a threatened abortion as half of these women will go on to miscarry. In most instances, fetal death occurs one to three weeks prior to the passage of conception products. In some instances, not all of the products will be expelled and surgical removal is necessary. Rarely, recurrent abortions occur, and anatomical, hormonal, and chromosomal abnormalities should be considered.

Cesarean Section

There are times when vaginal delivery of the fetus is not possible due to its size or position (Figure 18.2). There may also be circumstances in which the safety of the mother or fetus is dependent upon prompt delivery of the fetus, which can't be accomplished by vaginal delivery. In these instances, abdominal delivery via cesarean section (C-section) is indicated. This method of delivery is timely and can be done with spinal anesthesia in most cases. An incision through the lower abdomen and into the uterus enables the obstetrician to remove the fetus quickly from the uterus. Due to the risk of anesthesia, bleeding, infection, and longer recovery time, cesarean sections are reserved for those women with the problems mentioned above. Even so, nearly 25% of all deliveries are by cesarean section, but this num-

FIGURE 18.2
Breech presentation. A fetus in this position frequently cannot be delivered through the vagina.

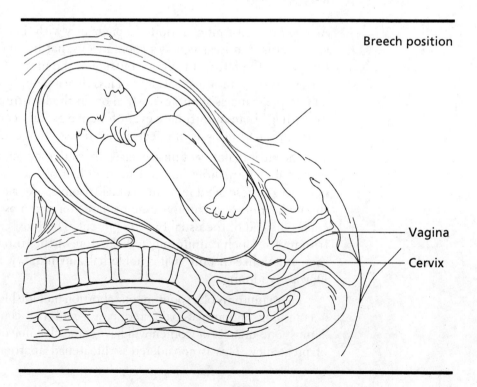

Breech position

Vagina

Cervix

ber may be decreasing as recent information reveals that women with a previous cesarean section can often safely attempt vaginal delivery.

Fetal Alcohol Syndrome

Alcohol consumption during pregnancy can result in infants with growth retardation, abnormal facial development, and central nervous system dysfunction. These problems may affect over 40% of children born to alcoholic mothers. The likelihood of having an infant with fetal alcohol syndrome depends on the amount of alcohol consumed. Even light to moderate drinkers have an increased risk of fetal alcohol syndrome, but their risk is lower than that of heavy drinkers. Stopping drinking at any time during the pregnancy improves the fetus's chance of normal development. Unfortunately, it is very difficult to differentiate between direct effects of alcohol on the fetus and compounding lifestyle factors of alcoholics (smoking, other drug use, and poor nutrition). These factors also influence the fetus, increasing the risk of abnormal development. Although no level of alcohol consumption is known to be safe during pregnancy, there are no clear-cut risks associated with an occasional drink.

Smoking, Caffeine, Illicit Drugs, and Aspartame in Pregnancy

Mothers who smoke during pregnancy have a higher rate of miscarriage, more premature births, and babies with decreased birth weight. There is also an increased risk of placental problems and complications with delivery. The risks of these complications for the mother and fetus increase with the number of cigarettes smoked. All women should be encouraged to stop smoking during pregnancy, and this is an opportune time to stop smoking completely.

Caffeine has not been shown to cause birth defects. Aspartame, an artificial sweetener marketed under the trade names NutraSweet and Equal, is used extensively in low-calorie products, especially diet soda beverages. Excessive amounts of aspartame have not been shown to cause birth defects, except possibly in mothers with a certain metabolic disease, phenylketonuria (PKU). In this disease, excessive amounts of aspartame may cause neurological problems in the fetus.

There is no documented increase in birth defects in mothers who use marijuana during pregnancy. Women who use cocaine during pregnancy have a much higher rate of miscarriages, more problems with the placenta, and babies with birth defects. There are more stillbirths and premature births, and newborns are smaller and have lower birth weights. Heroin addicts also have an increased risk of miscarriage and give births to infants that are premature, underdeveloped, and addicted to heroin. These infants can die from heroin withdrawal. Pregnant women on heroin should make every effort to enter a methadone program, and care should be taken that the fetus does not withdraw from narcotics in utero.

Infertility

Infertility is the inability to achieve pregnancy with repeated attempts at fertilization. Infertility has become more common as more women wait until an older age to have children and with the increased use of hormonal and mechanical birth control. If pregnancy is not achieved after one year of conscious effort to do so, then counseling may be indicated. After routine testing of each partner, 20% of couples will have no clear etiology of the infertility. In the remaining 80%, half are due to the female partner and half to the male.

Once the cause of infertility is determined, several treatment options are available to increase the likelihood of pregnancy. Hormonal manipulation, sperm concentrating techniques, surgery to correct anatomical obstruction to fertilization, artificial insemination, and even extra-utero fertilization are available. Extra-utero fertilization (the so-called "test tube baby" technique) involves obtaining an ovum surgically from the mother before ovulation and incubating of the extracted ovum with sperm. This is carried out in a media rich in nutritional elements to support the growth of the fetus until a time when it is implanted in the mother's uterus.

An interesting phenomenon has occurred as a result of infertility medications: increasing numbers of triplets, quadruplets, and quintuplets in the United States. This is due largely to the hormonal stimulation of several follicles instead of just one, so that more than one ovum is released with ovulation.

Birth Control

Birth control, or contraception, is the conscious effort to prevent pregnancy. Today, several types of contraception are available to suit individual lifestyles. Each type of contraception will be mentioned below with a short discussion of the mechanism of action. The table shows the actual effectiveness of these methods.

There are two methods of physiological ("natural") birth control. First, the withdrawal method involves removing the penis from the vagina before ejaculation occurs. This is also called *coitus interruptus* and is not very effective because the man may not know exactly when he will ejaculate, and even before ejaculation, some semen containing enough sperm to cause pregnancy may "leak" out. The second method is the *rhythm method* (natural family planning), or periodic abstinence. The woman charts her menstrual cycles, basal body temperature, and cervical mucus quality. Then, at the time during her cycle when fertilization is likely, complete abstinence from intercourse is practiced. With this method, nearly half of the menstrual cycle is off limits for intercourse. The effectiveness is similar to that of the withdrawal method.

There are several barrier methods of contraception. For their use to be effective, it is very important to follow directions. 1) *Spermicides* are chemicals that immobilize and kill sperm. They are available without a prescription and come in several forms (vaginal creams, foams, jellies, powders, and suppositories). They are only marginally effective when used alone, but when they are used in combination with other barrier methods, their effectiveness increases greatly. 2) The oldest and most commonly used barrier method is the male condom. A latex condom must be placed over an erect penis prior to intercourse, allowing enough space at the tip to contain the semen. It must be removed promptly after intercourse, intact, from the erect penis. Several condoms also contain a spermicide and are very effective if used appropriately. *Condoms are the only contraceptive method that help prevent the transmission of sexually transmitted diseases, including AIDS.* Condoms are 85% to 90% effective at preventing STDs and should always be used in addition to other forms of contraception for this reason. 3) The *diaphragm* and *cervical cap* are soft rubber cups that fit over the cervix and form a physical barrier to sperm. Spermicide should be used with each. The cervical cap fits more tightly, is more difficult to insert, but does not require frequent reapplication of additional spermicide as does the diaphragm. 4) The *contraceptive sponge* is a soft, synthetic object that blocks the cervix and releases spermicide. It is effective in the vagina for 24 hours and is available without a prescription.

Unlike barrier methods of contraception, long-term methods free the individual from the responsibility of birth control with each sexual encounter. There are two types of long-term contraception. First, the *intrauterine device* (IUD) is a plastic object that contains copper or progesterone. It is inserted into the uterus by a physician and remains in place for up to three years. It prevents implantation, probably by irritating the uterus. The second long-term method is *contraceptive implants* (Norplant). These capsules contain progestin, which is slowly released when implanted under the skin of the upper arm. Insertion of the capsules is relatively easy, but removing them can be difficult due to excessive scar formation around the capsules. Efficacy of the implants is dependent on body habitus and are less effective in obese women. Both the IUD and contraceptive implants are reversible when removed.

Oral contraceptives, or birth control pills, are composed of estrogen and progestin hormones that prevent ovulation. The pills must be taken daily during the first 21 days of the cycle. They are then stopped to allow menstrual bleeding to occur. Some side effects are associated with oral contraceptives. They can usually be controlled by changing the dose or type of hormone combination. *Women using oral contraception should not smoke.* Smoking markedly increases the risk of stroke, blood clots, and heart attacks, especially in women over 35 years of age.

Surgical sterilization is available for men and women. In women, a *tubal ligation* involves "tying" the fallopian tubes. This can be performed with laproscopic surgery but requires general anesthesia. It is sometimes performed following delivery. A *vasectomy* is the removal of a portion of the vas deferens. This procedure can be done with a local anesthetic in a physician's office. Both forms of sterilization should be considered permanent, although it may be possible to "reverse" the procedure in some cases.

Methods of Birth Control

Method	Effectiveness
Physiological	
Rhythm	76%
Withdrawal	77%
Barrier†	
Spermicides‡	80%
Condom	90%
Diaphragm	80%
Cervical cap	90%
Sponge	90%
Long-term	
Intrauterine device	95%
Implants	99%
Oral contraception	98%
Permanent	
Vasectomy	99.9%
Tubal ligation	99.9%
None	15%

†when used with spermicides
‡spermicides used alone

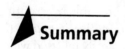

Summary

Healthy pregnancy and fetal development are dependent on a host of factors. It is the mother's responsibility to avoid substances or conditions known to increase risk to the fetus. Proper prenatal care does not always ensure a healthy delivery, but many of the risks can be reduced.

Selection of contraception is a personal choice based on lifestyle and motivation. Taking a pill each day may be more feasible than use of a barrier method, which requires pre-intercourse preparation. Couples who do not want children or have the desired number of children may elect permanent surgical sterilization. Individual choices about contraception must be respected by the physician and the sexual partner(s).

19 Prevention and Health Maintenance

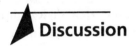

Discussion

Although advances in medical research and technology have led to improved treatment of diseases and prolonged survival, the key to a healthy life lies in the prevention of disease. Genetic factors play a large role in the risk of developing disease, and exposure to infections or traumatic injury cannot always be avoided. However, certain steps can be taken to improve your health and prevent certain "lifestyle diseases."

Nutrition

Nutrition has gained attention in the medical profession as new information has become available supporting the significant impact diet can have on health. Several debilitating diseases are caused by improper diet or can be prevented by changes in diet. A balanced diet provides not only adequate calories but also the important vitamins and minerals necessary for growth, development, and continuing body function. Calcium and iron are two minerals that are generally lacking in American diets. Iron prevents the development of anemia, and adequate calcium decreases the risk of osteoporosis. Likewise, too much of some things in the diet may be undesirable. Persons with risk factors for atherosclerosis may benefit from decreasing the amount of cholesterol and saturated fats in the diet.

Diseases of caloric intake can involve either excessive or inadequate ingestion. Obesity is a common problem in the United States and contributes to other medical disorders. The underlying problem is a mathematical one in which caloric intake exceeds energy expenditure and the result is weight gain. Rarely is there an underlying metabolic cause that can easily be reversed. *Anorexia nervosa* and *bulimia* are two problems involving a lack of calories. Persons with anorexia "starve" themselves by not eating, and bulimics exhibit "binge and purge" behavior in which vomiting is induced after eating. These disorders are common among young women and stem from problems with body self-image.

Cancer and Nutrition

It appears that both individual genetic characteristics and environmental factors play a role in cancer. Although tobacco is the major environmental factor associated with cancer, certain dietary factors may also be involved. Unfortunately, it has been quite difficult to prove that certain diets or dietary products cause or prevent a certain type of cancer. It is unethical to conduct a study in which potentially harmful food products are given to a group of healthy subjects in order to assess whether they develop cancer more frequently than people on other diets. Much of the information on nutrition and cancer is from studies that analyze differences between large populations with markedly different diets. Information may also be gained when a portion of a population adopts a new diet. For example, a large number of Japanese who moved to California have been studied. There is more stomach cancer and less colon and breast cancer among Japanese living in Japan than among Americans. However, in Japanese who have moved to California, the rate of colon and breast cancer has increased, while the incidence of stomach cancer has remained constant. This suggests (but does not prove) that environmental factors are contributing to the rise in breast and colon cancer. A major contribution may have been a change in diet. A second large population that has been studied is Seventh-Day Adventists, a religious group that consumes a vegetarian diet and abstains from alcohol and tobacco. The incidence of tobacco-related and alcohol-related cancers are decreased in this group. In addition, other cancers that are thought to be related to diet are reduced in this group.

Based on these and other studies, the American Cancer Society has made the following recommendations: (1) Avoid obesity. The incidence of breast, gallbladder, and gynecological cancers are increased in obese people, especially females. (2) Decrease total fat intake. Diets high in fat may be related to increased risks of breast and colon cancer. (3) Increase high-fiber foods. Dietary fiber may reduce the risk of colon cancer by increasing stool bulk, changing the transit time of intestinal contents, modifying bile in the intestine, or altering intestinal bacteria; all of these factors have been implicated in colon cancer. (4) Include foods containing vitamins A and C. These vitamins may have some connection with preventing colon, bladder, lung, esophagus, and stomach cancer. (5) Consume cruciferous vegetables such as cauliflower, cabbage, and broccoli. These foods are high in fiber and in vitamins A and C, and they appear to reduce the incidence of colon cancer in animal studies, an effect that may be due to the large amounts of *indoles* in these foods. (6) Consume alcoholic beverages only in moderate amounts. Alcohol has been associated with cancers of the liver, upper digestive tract, and breasts. (7) Consume smoked, salt-cured, and nitrite-cured foods only in moderate amounts. These foods have been associated with cancers of the esophagus and stomach.

In summary, attempts to link diet with cancer should be viewed with caution, and much remains to be learned about the possible connections between nutrition and cancer. Nonetheless, many cancer researchers believe that enough information is known already to recommend some or all of the above guidelines, especially since they carry no risks.

Cholesterol

The cholesterol problem is complicated by several factors. For example, cholesterol metabolism is determined genetically to a large extent. Some persons ingesting high-cholesterol diets have normal blood cholesterol levels, and others on low-cholesterol diets have dangerously high blood cholesterol levels. Because cholesterol metabolism is specific to the individual, mass treatment or analysis of this problem may be inappropriate. Another complication of the cholesterol problem is that hypercholesterolemia, or elevated blood cholesterol, is a silent "disease" and cannot be detected without a blood test. An individual may feel great while cholesterol plaques are accumulating in the arteries. Although it may be inappropriate for everyone to be screened for elevated cholesterol, it is sensible for people at risk for cardiovascular disease to have their cholesterol levels checked. People at risk for cardiovascular disease include those with a family history of such problems, those who smoke, and those with hypertension, diabetes, or obesity. If elevated blood cholesterol is discovered, the problem may respond to dietary changes, weight loss, and exercise; these measures are desirable ways of treating the condition, because they eliminate the need for medications. However, lifestyle changes are not effective in everyone with elevated cholesterol. In these people, medications may be indicated. Also, because factors such as smoking and hypertension usually contribute more to cardiovascular disease than does elevated cholesterol, checking and treating hypertension and the cessation of smoking are at least as important in prolonging life in some people as is decreasing the cholesterol level in the blood.

To summarize, cholesterol is an individual problem. Some people clearly benefit from cholesterol reduction, although medications instead of or in addition to dietary changes may be required to achieve the reduction. People who have coronary artery disease or have had coronary bypass surgery, for example, benefit from cholesterol reduction, and it is sensible for them to check their cholesterol levels and treat them if necessary. It is sensible for people at high risk for cardiovascular disease to be screened for cholesterol levels due to the silent nature of the problem. In these individuals, screening and treating hypertension and cessation of smoking are also important. Because cholesterol levels in some people do not respond to changes in diet and lifestyle, blood cholesterol should be measured *before* changes in diet and lifestyle are undertaken. If blood cholesterol is checked only after dietary changes are made, it is impossible to determine whether the dietary change has lowered the cholesterol level.

Alcohol

Ten to 15 million people in the United States have an alcohol addiction or a dependency on alcohol. Alcoholism is a condition in which repeated problems are caused by alcohol addiction. There are multiple, complex causes of this disease. Alcoholism consumes a large percentage of health care resources and causes many social, emotional, occupational, and educational problems.

Alcohol abuse contributes to many medical problems. Liver cirrhosis, pancreatitis, peptic ulcers, and liver cancer are caused by alcohol. Neurological problems are common and include blackout spells, memory loss, peripheral neurological dysfunction, and problems with balance and gait. Malnutrition is a huge problem among alcoholics because it leads to poorer health, predisposes to disease, and impairs the healing process. An enlarged heart with decreased function and hypertension are caused by alcohol. The hematological effects of alcohol include anemia and bleeding complications due to liver disease.

Alcoholism is not a hopeless disease. As many as 70% of alcoholics can stop drinking with appropriate help, although this will be a lifelong endeavor. Many alcohol-related diseases will resolve when one stops drinking, but some diseases are not reversible once the damage has been done. A final mention of fetal alcohol syndrome (see Chapter 18) will be made because of its devastating effect on an infant with no control of its alcohol exposure.

Smoking

Tobacco abuse has been declining in the United States, but the number of teenage smokers has risen. Smoking increases one's risk of disease and decreases life expectancy. The risk of death and disease is proportional to the total number of cigarettes smoked in a lifetime ("pack-years," discussed in Chapter 14). Smoking increases the risks of cancer, especially lung cancer. It also contributes to cancer of the mouth, throat, esophagus, kidney, bladder, pancreas, and uterus. Chronic lung diseases (emphysema and chronic bronchitis) are markedly increased among smokers. Actually, the risk of lung cancer and disease is ten times higher in smokers than nonsmokers. The risk of developing atherosclerosis (in coronary or peripheral vessels) and peptic ulcer disease is also higher in smokers. The risks of smoking during pregnancy was mentioned in Chapter 18.

Fortunately, the risks associated with smoking decrease after quitting. The risk of cardiovascular disease returns to normal in three to five years after quitting. If cancer and chronic lung disease have not developed, the risks for these diseases is normal in seven to ten years. Quitting is a difficult task, even for a highly motivated individual. In addition to behavior modification, medication to control the side effects of withdrawal and various forms of nicotine (gum, patch, and, soon, a nasal spray) are available under medical supervision. The nicotine substitutes are used temporarily to satisfy the craving for nicotine and should not be used in combination with cigarettes. The most effective way to deal with smoking is never to start.

Exercise

Aerobic exercise has been shown to decrease the risk of cardiovascular disease. Aerobic exercise (walking, jogging, cycling, swimming, tennis, aerobics) for 20 to 30 minutes at least three times a week is recommended. Weight-bearing exercises (not swimming or cycling) and weight-lifting exercises prevent osteoporosis (bone loss). A combination of these two types of exercise can help prevent debilitating disease as well as improve self-image and confidence.

Health Care Maintenance

Health care maintenance is the investment in routine examinations and screening studies for the prevention or early detection. The concept of keeping healthy by regular checkups instead of just treating diseases once they become symptomatic has changed the approach to health care. Varying guidelines has been established by medical organizations; the general recommendations are listed below:

Blood pressure check—every 2 years
Cholesterol screening—every 5 years beginning in the 20s
Pap smear—every year once sexually active; if three consecutive normal tests, every 2 to 3 years
Tetanus immunization booster—every 10 years
Influenza immunization—yearly starting at age 65
Breast self-exam—monthly
Clinical breast exam—every 3 years, then yearly after age 39
Mammography—baseline study at age 35 to 40; every 2 years from 41 to 50, then yearly
Testicular self-exam—monthly
Clinical testicular exam—yearly
Stool test for blood—yearly starting at age 50
Endoscope of distal colon—every three years starting at age 50

The above list is appropriate only for individuals who are asymptomatic and do not have risk factors for certain diseases. Once a positive screening test is obtained, future tests are not for "screening" purposes but for follow-up and diagnosis and should be done when deemed appropriated by the physician. Although preventive measures are made available by healthcare professionals, each individual should take responsibility for his or her own health. This is done by routinely performing self-examinations and seeking medical care for screening evaluations. With these efforts, a longer, healthier life is ahead.

Glossary

ABORTION—spontaneous or elective termination of a pregnancy prior to fetal viability

ACNE—an inflammatory process of the skin caused by buildup of sebum, bacteria, and dead cells in hair follicles, leading to pustules or comedones

ACROMEGALY—a condition secondary to overproduction of growth hormone resulting in enlargement of bones in the face, hands, and feet

ACUTE—of illness, having a short course

ADAPTIVE RESPONSES—the body's ability to heal or compensate for diseases

AIDS (acquired immunodeficiency syndrome)—diseases characterized by a compromised immune system and opportunistic infections, such as pneumocystis carnii, lymphoma, and Kaposi's sarcoma; caused by the human immunodeficiency virus (HIV); transmitted by blood, or bodily fluids, and sexual contact

ALLERGEN—a substance causing an allergic response

ALLERGY—an acquired hypersensitivity to a substance that does not usually cause a reaction

AMENORRHEA—lack of menstrual bleeding

AMPUTATION—removal of a part of the body, such as a toe or an arm

AMYLASE—enzyme that metabolizes starch; produced by the pancreas

ANAPHYLAXIS—a systemic, widespread allergic reaction that can lead to death without prompt emergency treatment

ANEMIA—decreased red blood cell concentration in the blood

ANEURYSM—dilation, or enlargement, of an artery

ANGINA—chest discomfort caused by inadequate blood flow to the heart muscle

ANGIOGRAM—study to diagnose and define the location and extent of an arterial blockage by injecting a radio-opaque dye

ANTIBIOTIC—a chemical compound that kills or prevents growth of organisms

ANTIBODY—a protein substance produced by the body to respond to an antigen

ANTIGEN—a substance that induces the formation of antibodies

APPENDICITIS—an infection of the appendix

157

ARTERIOVENOUS MALFORMATION—abnormal arterial-venous connection, completely bypassing the capillaries

ARTHRALGIA—pain in the joints, sometimes due to inflammation

ARTHRITIS—inflammation of one or more joints

ARTHROSCOPIC SURGERY—a technique to examine and treat joint disorders by inserting a small, fiber-optic scope through a skin incision

ASCITES—accumulation of fluid in the peritoneal cavity

ASTHMA—disorder characterized by intermittent wheezing, chest tightness, and cough with variable airflow obstruction and inflammation

ATHEROSCLEROSIS—disease in which cholesterol plaques build up in arteries causing a narrowing of the vessel lumen

ATRIAL FIBRILLATION—heartbeat caused by irregular atrial rhythm

ATRIAL SEPTAL DEFECT—a congenital opening between the right and left atria of the heart

AUTOIMMUNE DISEASES—disorders in which the body makes antibodies that attack its own tissue

BACTERIA—microorganisms that may cause disease

BASAL BODY TEMPERATURE—temperature upon awakening; recorded daily to help determine time of ovulation

BASAL CELL EPITHELIOMA—tumor of the basal cells of the skin

BENIGN—mild or nonmalignant

BENIGN PROSTATIC HYPERTROPHY—enlargement of the prostate that typically occurs with aging; may lead to obstruction of the urethra and difficulty voiding

BILIRUBIN—a product of hemoglobin breakdown, processed by the liver

BONE MARROW TRANSPLANTATION—the placing of compatible, healthy, donor bone marrow into patients with various diseases, such as leukemia and other cancers. The recipients' own bone marrow must first be destroyed. In autologous transplantation, the bone marrow is harvested from the patient during a time of remission.

BREAST CANCER—common cancer that, if found early, may be curable with surgery, medication, radiation, or a combination of them

BREECH PRESENTATION—situation in which a fetus is not in the usual head-down position at the time of delivery.; often requires a cesarean section

BRONCHITIS—an infection of the mucosa of the bronchi

BRONCHOSCOPY—a procedure using a fiber-optic scope to visualize the trachea and bronchi and obtain a biopsy of the lung parenchyma, if indicated

BURSA—a sac around a joint, filled with synovial fluid, that acts as a buffer in areas of friction in the body

BURSITIS—an inflammation of the sac (bursa) surrounding a joint, usually characterized by pain, heat, and swelling

CALLUS—connective tissue and cartilage that develops from the procallus in fracture healing. This stabilizes the fracture site to a great extent. The callus calcifies, and final bone remodeling occurs.

CARDIOLOGIST—a physician who specializes in the study and treatment of heart disease

CARDIOTHORACIC SURGEON—a surgeon who specializes in the surgical treatment of heart and lung disease

CARPAL TUNNEL SYNDROME—the entrapment of the median nerve in the carpal tunnel of the wrist

CATARACT—opacity of the lens or cornea

CAT SCAN (computerized axial tomography)—radiologic technique used to show detailed images of a tissue in a transverse plane

CEREBRAL VASCULAR ACCIDENT (CVA)—a neurological event caused by inadequate blood supply to an area of the brain

CERVICAL CANCER—cancer of the cervix, linked to exposure to human papilloma virus, early sexual relations, and multiple sexual partners

CERVICAL CAP—small rubber-like cap that fits over the cervix to prevent conception; must be fitted by a physician and does not protect from sexually transmitted diseases

CERVICAL DYSPLASIA—changes in the cells of the cervix, found on a Pap smear, that are usually precancerous lesions

CESAREAN SECTION—delivery of a fetus through the abdomen

CHEMOTHERAPY—the treatment of disease with chemicals or pharmacological agents

CHLAMYDIA—microorganism causing a wide variety of illnesses, including genital infections (STD), pneumonia, and conjunctivitis

CHOLESTEROL—a chemical found throughout the body, important in metabolism; contributes to the development of atherosclerosis when elevated in the blood

CHRONIC—of illness, having a long course

CIRRHOSIS—chronic disease of the liver with structural changes and impaired function

CLAUDICATION—pain in the legs from decreased oxygen delivery secondary to cholesterol plaques

COITUS INTERRUPTUS—withdrawal of the penis from the vagina prior to ejaculation

COLONOSCOPY—examination of the lower gastrointestinal tract utilizing a fiber-optic scope

COLPOSCOPY—the visualization of the vulva, vagina, and cervix through a specialized microscope during a pelvic exam

COMEDONES—discolored dried sebum plugging a skin follicle

CONDOM—thin, flexible sheath worn over the penis; used to help prevent pregnancy and transmission of sexual diseases

CONJUNCTIVITIS—infection of the conjunctiva caused by virus or bacteria

CONTACT DERMATITIS—an inflammatory reaction of the skin that develops after contact with an allergen, resulting in itching and redness; commonly caused by poison ivy or poison oak

CONTRACEPTIVE IMPLANTS—small, flexible capsules inserted into the upper arm that slowly release progestin for contraception up to five years; must be inserted by a physician; completely reversible after removal

CONTRACEPTIVE SPONGE—synthetic device inserted prior to intercourse to help prevent pregnancy by releasing spermicide and covering the cervix

CRYOTHERAPY—freezing of tissue, usually with liquid nitrogen; often used in the treatment of cervical dysplasia and warts.

CYSTIC FIBROSIS—a hereditary disease in which the exocrine glands of the body secrete abnormally thick mucus; involves the lungs and the pancreas

CYSTOSCOPY—examination of the bladder and ureters with a fiber-optic scope

DEBRIDEMENT—removal of dead skin

DEMENTIA—the progressive deterioration of mental and cognitive function.

DERMATOLOGY—the study of disorders of the skin

DIAGNOSIS—the recognition or determination of the nature of a disease based on physical examination, history of the illness, and any specialized tests (blood, x-ray, etc.) deemed necessary

DIALYSIS—the separation of solute molecules via a selectively permeable membrane; used to clear the blood of harmful metabolites in kidney failure; may be done through the blood by hemodialysis or through the abdomen via peritoneal dialysis

DIAPHRAGM—a flexible rubber contraceptive object inserted into the vagina to cover the cervix prior to intercourse; must be left in place after intercourse at least six hours

DIARRHEA—frequent passage of unformed, watery stools

DISEASE—a disruption in the body's ability to function normally

DISLOCATION—the displacement of a joint from its usual anatomic position

DYSMENORRHEA—painful menses, or menstrual cramps

DYSURIA—painful urination

ECHOCARDIOGRAPHY—an ultrasound technique to examine the heart, and blood flow through it

ECTOPIC PREGNANCY—a pregnancy occurring anywhere other than the uterus, most commonly in the fallopian tubes (tubular pregnancy); a surgical emergency

ELECTROCARDIOGRAM—a recording of the electrical activity of the heart using electrodes placed on the skin

ELECTROENCEPHALOGRAM (EEG)—a tracing of the electrical activity of the brain using electrodes placed on the scalp

EMBOLUS—mass of undissolved matter in the blood or lymphatic system; usually a blood clot

EMPHYSEMA—a disease in which the alveolar structure breaks down, resulting in the loss of functional lung parenchyma and leading to hypoxemia and air trapping

ENDOCRINOLOGIST—a physician specializing in the study and treatment of the endocrine system

ENDOMETRIAL CANCER—cancer of the lining of the uterus, more commonly found in postmenopausal women. Abnormal bleeding is a common symptom.

ENDOSCOPY—examination of an internal body area utilizing a fiber-optic scope

EQUILIBRIUM—state of balance

ERYTHROPOIETIN—a hormone produced by the kidney to stimulate red blood cell formation

ESTROGEN—"female" sex hormone; responsible for the development of secondary sexual characteristics and for cyclic changes of the vagina and uterus

FETAL ALCOHOL SYNDROME—birth defects caused by chronic alcohol use during pregnancy

FIBER-OPTIC SCOPE—flexible glass or plastic device that transmits light by internal reflections from fibers; can be used to visualize internal structures

FOLEY CATHETER—a flexible rubber tube inserted into the bladder through the urethra in order to drain urine

FRACTURE—a break of bone or cartilage

GALLSTONES—rock-like substance, usually formed of cholesterol, that develops in the gallbladder

GANGRENE—death of tissue, usually due to insufficient blood supply

GASTROENTERITIS—an infection of the stomach or intestine caused by viruses or bacteria, with nausea, vomiting, and diarrhea as the most common symptoms

GASTROENTROLOGIST—a physician specializing in the study of the gastrointestinal system and associated organs

GASTRO-ESOPHOGEAL REFLUX—the reflux of stomach contents into the esophagus

GENITAL WARTS—warts in the genital area caused by human papilloma virus

GLAUCOMA—disease of the eye resulting from high intraocular pressure; may lead to blindness

GOITER—a benign or malignant enlargement of the thyroid gland

GONORRHEA—a sexually transmitted disease causing infection of internal sexual organs; frequently asymptomatic

GOUT—a hereditary disorder of uric acid metabolism, frequently causing arthritic attacks, commonly of the great toe

GUILLAIN-BARRÉ SYNDROME—a disease involving demyelination of the neuronal axons, characterized by a progressive loss of motor function

GYNECOLOGIST—a physician who specializes in the study and treatment of the female reproductive system

HEART ATTACK (myocardial infarction)—a disorder in which blood flow to an area of the heart ceases, leading to tissue death

HEMATOLOGIST—physician who studies and treats disorders of the blood

HEMATURIA—blood in the urine; may be microscopic or gross (visible to the naked eye)

HEMOPHILIA—hereditary disorder in which a factor in the clotting cascade is lacking

HEPATITIS—inflammation of the liver caused by a variety of agents, including viral and bacterial agents

HERPES SIMPLEX VIRUS—organism causing painful, blister-like sores of the skin of the genitals and mouth

HORMONE—a substance produced by one part of the body, such as a gland, which produces an effect on another part of the body

HYPERCHOLESTEROLEMIA—elevated cholesterol in the blood

HYPEROPIA—far-sightedness

HYPERTENSION—an elevation in blood pressure, generally considered to be a systolic pressure (top number) greater than 140 mm Hg and a diastolic pressure (bottom number) greater than 90 mm Hg

HYPOXEMIA—low oxygen content in the blood, resulting in poor oxygen delivery to the tissues

HYSTERECTOMY—surgical removal of the uterus (does not mean automatic removal of the ovaries)

IMMUNIZATION—administrating of an immunogen in order to develop protection from a disease

IMPETIGO—a highly contagious bacterial infection of the skin caused by staphylococcal or streptococcal bacteria

IMPOTENCE—the inability to achieve or maintain an erection; may be physiological or psychological in origin

INCONTINENCE—inability to control the flow of urine

INFARCTION—an area of tissue that dies following cessation of blood supply

INFECTION—a condition in which a pathologic agent (bacterium, virus) multiplies and produces injury

INFERTILITY—the inability to conceive after repeated attempts

INTRAUTERINE DEVICE (IUD)—copper or hormone-releasing device inserted into the uterus by a physician to prevent pregnancy

ISCHEMIA—local and temporary insufficient blood supply

JAUNDICE—a yellow discoloration of the skin and eyes due to increased bilirubin and primarily caused by liver disease

JOINT ASPIRATION—the removal of fluid from a joint using a needle and syringe; may be both diagnostic and therapeutic

LAPROSCOPIC SURGERY—surgery performed in the abdomen using a fiber-optic light and small surgical instruments

LARYNGITIS—an infection of the vestibular and true vocal cords leading to hoarseness and loss of voice

LEUKEMIA—acute or chronic disease, sometimes fatal, characterized by uncontrolled growth of leukocytes and their precursors

LIPASE—a fat-splitting enzyme

LIPIDS—a group of fats or fat-like substances, including fatty acids and cholesterol

LITHOTRIPSY—a procedure using shock waves to break up kidney stones and, sometimes, gallstones

LOCAL—confined to one location or organ

LUMBAR PUNCTURE—a procedure in which a needle is passed between the lumbar vertebra into the spinal canal to collect cerebrospinal fluid for analysis

LYMPHOMA—a solid tumor composed of lymphocytes proliferating in lymphatic tissue

MACULAR DEGENERATION—degradation of the macula of the eye, commonly occurring in the elderly

MALIGNANCY—a tumor or neoplasm that is cancerous

MALNUTRITION—lack of necessary food substances from improper intake or incomplete absorption

MAMMOGRAPHY—a special radiological examination of the breast tissue to look for cancer

MARFAN'S SYNDROME—an inherited disease of the collagen fibers of the body

MELANOMA—a malignant, potentially fatal skin cancer arising from the pigment-producing cells (melanocytes) of the skin

MENINGITIS—an infection of the meninges and the cerebrospinal fluid

MENOPAUSE—cessation of reproductive function in women

METABOLISM—all energy and material transformations that occur within an organism

METASTASIS—the spread of cancer from one area of the body to another

MIGRAINE HEADACHE—paroxysmal headache, often unilateral and accompanied by light sensitivity, nausea, and vomiting

MISCARRIAGE—spontaneous abortion of a pregnancy prior to the second trimester

MITTELSCHMERZ—a pain or sensation in the lower abdomen indicating rupture of a follicle during ovulation

MULTIPLE SCLEROSIS—a disease caused by the destruction of the myelin sheaths that encase the neurons and leading to nerve conduction abnormalities

MURMUR—abnormal heart sound caused by blood passing the heart valves

MUSCULAR DYSTROPHY—an inherited disease of the muscle fibers leading to profound weakness and death

MYASTHENIA GRAVIS—a disease in which the body produces antibodies to the acetylcholine receptors

MYOPIA—near-sightedness

NEPHROLOGIST—a physician specializing in the medical treatment and study of the kidney and bladder

NEUROLOGIST—a physician specializing in the study and treatment of the nervous system

NEUROSURGEON—a physician who specializes in operations on the brain, spinal cord, peripheral and central nerves, and vertebral column

OBESITY—excess amount of fat on the body; generally considered to be more than 20% to 30% above average weight

OBSTETRICIAN—a physician who specializes in pregnancy and delivery of babies

ONCOLOGIST—a physician who specializes in the treatment and study of cancer

OPHTHALMOLOGIST—a physician who specializes in the study and treatment of eye diseases

OPTOMETRIST—a person trained to examine eyes to test for and prescribe lenses for visual acuity

ORAL CONTRACEPTIVES (birth control pills)—small doses of hormones, usually estrogen and progestin, taken orally; interfere with ovulation and thus prevent pregnancy

ORTHOPEDIC SURGEON—physician who specializes in problems affecting the bone, joints, and musculature

OSTEOARTHRITIS—the "wear and tear" arthritis that occurs with the degeneration of the joints with age

OSTEOPOROSIS—reduction in density or quantity of bone, usually occurring in postmenopausal women or elderly men. Smoking, alcohol use, poor dietary habits and hereditary factors also contribute to the development of osteoporosis.

OTITIS EXTERNA—infection of the external auditory canal, commonly caused by fungus

OTITIS MEDIA—infection of the middle ear, caused by viruses or bacteria

PACEMAKER—an electrical device, consisting of a battery-operated generator and one or two wires, designed to stimulate the heart

PANCREATITIS—inflammation of the pancreas

PAP SMEAR—a test, developed by George Papanicolaou, to detect cancer and precancerous lesions, commonly of the cervix, utilizing a specialized staining technique

PARAPLEGIA—the paralysis or paresis of the lower extremities, often the result of a spinal cord injury

PATHOGEN—any agent that causes disease

PEPTIC ULCER DISEASE—excess acid and pepsin production in the stomach leading to ulcer disease

PET SCAN (positron emission tomography)—a specialized radiographic technique providing information about blood supply and metabolic activity

PHANTOM PAIN—sensation of pain or feeling in a limb that has been removed

PHYSIATRIST—physicians who specialize in rehabilitation

PNEUMONIA—a lower respiratory tract infection

PNEUMOTHORAX—the presence of air in the pleural cavity, usually the result of trauma

PREMENSTRUAL SYNDROME—a collection of emotional, physical, and mental symptoms occurring prior to the onset of menses

PROCALLUS—the first stage of fracture healing; formed by the blood clot around the fractured segments

PRODROME—a symptom indicative of an impending illness

PROGESTERONE—a "female" hormone important in the second half of the menstrual cycle and in development of the placenta and mammary glands

PROGNOSIS—an educated prediction of the outcome of the disease and potential complications arising from it

PROSTAGLANDINS—a group of biologically active substances within the body that act as local modulators of tissue biochemical reactions

PROSTHESIS—a constructed substitute for a missing or diseased part, such as a limb or heart valve

PSORIASIS—a chronic, common skin disorder characterized by rough, scaling plaques

QUADRIPLEGIA—paralysis of all four extremities, often the result of a spinal cord injury in the cervical neck region

RADIATION—ionizing rays used for diagnostic or therapeutic purposes

RADIATION THERAPY—use of ionizing radiation in the treatment of malignant neoplasms

RENAL CELL CARCINOMA—cancer arising from the renal tubules

RESTRICTIVE LUNG DISEASES—disorders causing decreased volume capacity secondary to loss of airspace units or the inability to expand the lungs

RHEUMATOID ARTHRITIS—an autoimmune disorder that eventually leads to the buildup of inflamed joint tissue that can destroy the joint

RHEUMATOLOGIST—a physician who studies and treats diseases of the joints, connective tissues, and immune system

RHINITIS—an inflammation of the nasal mucosa

RHYTHM METHOD—means of family planning that avoids sexual intercourse during fertile periods, utilizing cervical mucus, basal body temperature, and charting of menses

SEBACEOUS GLAND—oil-secreting gland of the skin

SEBUM—fatty secretion from the sebaceous glands of the skin

SEIZURE DISORDER—a disease resulting from disorganized, electrical brain discharges manifested by uncontrollable, random, and sporadic motor, sensory or mental activity

SEXUALLY TRANSMITTED DISEASES (STDs)—infections passed between partners during sexual activity

SHINGLES—disease caused by a resurgence of the herpes zoster virus (chicken pox virus) and causing painful red blisters along a dermatone

SINUSITIS—an infection of the lining of the sinuses

SLIPPED DISC—herniated nucleus pulposis of the vertebral canal; may cause neurological impairment

SPECULUM—metal or plastic instrument used for examining canals, such as the vagina

SPERMICIDES—chemicals that kill sperm

SPRAIN—injury resulting from a partial or complete tear of the ligaments or tendons supporting a joint structure

SQUAMOUS CELL CARCINOMA—cancer of the squamous cell of the skin

STRAIN—a minor injury caused by overstretching a muscle or tendon

STRATUM CORNEUM—outermost layer of the epidermis

STRESS FRACTURE—small disruption in the bone structure that results from repetitive impact, as in running or jumping

SYMPTOM—an alteration in sensation, appearance, or function; used in the diagnosis of diseases

SYPHILIS—a sexually transmitted disease that initially causes a painless genital ulcer; can become systemic

SYSTEMIC DISEASE—disease involving several organs throughout the body

TENDONITIS—an inflammation of a tendon, as in tennis elbow

TESTOSTERONE—an androgen hormone, produced by the testes, that promotes growth of secondary sexual characteristics and occurrence of erections

TETANUS—a severe disease, caused by the bacterium *Clostridium tetani*, that produces a toxin leading to the blocking of the inhibitory neurons of the motor system, resulting in increased and uncontrolled motor tone

THROMBOLYTIC THERAPY—a medication that dissolves a blood clot, leading to restoration of blood flow; commonly used in heart attacks

THROMBOPHLEBITIS—inflammation of a vein that occurs with the formation of a thrombus

THROMBUS—a blood clot that obstructs a blood vessel

TRICHOMONAS—sexually transmitted flagellate parasite causing itching and yellow, foamy vaginal discharge

TRIGLYCERIDES—fatty substances found in the blood

TUBAL LIGATION—permanent surgical closing of the fallopian tubes with clips, electrocoagualtion, or sutures

TUMOR—a swelling or growth

ULCER—a shallow, erosive sore caused by some form of trauma

ULTRASOUND—use of inaudible sound frequencies to outline shapes of various tissues or organs

UPPER RESPIRATORY INFECTION—a disease, usually viral and self-limited, of the upper airways, nose, and throat

URINARY TRACT INFECTION—an infection of the urethra or bladder

UROLOGIST—a physician (surgeon) specializing in the kidney and bladder

URTICARIA—vascular reaction of the skin causing pale, itching wheals, usually caused by some irritant or allergen

VARICOSE VEINS—enlarged, twisted superficial veins, commonly found in the legs

VASECTOMY—surgical severance of the vas deferens to prevent sperm transport into the ejaculate

VENTILATOR—a mechanical method of delivering air to a patient via an endotracheal tube and mechanical pump

VENTRICULAR SEPTAL DEFECT—congenital opening between the right and left ventricle

VIRUS—a minute organism that is totally dependent on cell nutrients for reproductive and metabolic needs

WART—a skin elevation resulting from hypertrophy of the epidermis caused by a papillomavirus

WILM'S TUMOR—a form of renal cancer, found in children, composed of many types of tissues, including bone, muscle, epithelium, and cartilage